DELICIOUS CARNIVORE DIET RECIPES FOR BEGINNERS:

Easy weight loss with complete day-by-day cooking plans

By PHYLIS .R. STOVALL

ACKNOWLEDGMENT

Table of Contents

Synopsis of the carnivore diet theory

Individual encounters or reasons for researching the carnivorous diet

Purpose of the book

Synopsis of the carnivore diet theory

The carnivore diet is a way of thinking about food and health that is rooted in our ancestral roots, rather than only focusing on what you consume. Imagine our hunter-gatherer ancestors depending on the abundance of land to survive. They did not have aisles upon aisles of fruits and vegetables or stores filled with prepackaged goods. Rather, they survived on the flesh and other animal items that they could hunt and gather.

The core of the carnivore diet philosophy is to embrace our primitive inclinations and fuel our bodies with the same foods that provided generations of sustenance for our ancestors. It's about returning to the essentials, streamlining our diets, and re-establishing our relationship with the foods that nature offers.

However, it's an attitude as much as a diet. It involves accepting the belief that animal products can feed our bodies with all they need to survive and rejecting the contemporary view that we need a wide range of meals to be healthy. It's about challenging received knowledge and investigating alternate dietary and health regimens.

The fundamental principle of the carnivore diet is to minimize or completely eliminate plant-based meals in favor of animal foods that are high in nutrients. This entails avoiding most fruits, vegetables, grains, and legumes and concentrating on meat, fish, eggs, and other animal products. It is a significant shift from the normal Western diet, which places a strong emphasis on plant-based foods as the cornerstone of a balanced diet.

Why, therefore, would someone decide to eat in this manner? Regaining one's health and energy is important to many. They could have suffered from stomach troubles, long-term medical illnesses, or weight difficulties, and switching to a carnivorous diet helped them feel better. They wish to educate others about the transformative impact of an animal-based diet, having personally experienced it themselves.

Some are drawn to the carnivore diet because of its clarity and simplicity. In a world where dietary recommendations appear to change every day and food labels are replete with technicalities, the concept of consuming just meat and animal products may be surprisingly simple. It's a return to the fundamentals, a natural and instinctual method of eating.

The carnivore diet is mostly about reestablishing our relationship with nature, however, that may not be the most significant point. It's about acknowledging the importance of the creatures that support us and the significant influence that our dietary decisions have on the world, the ecosystem, and our own health. This eating style honors sustainability, simplicity, and the body's inherent intelligence.

The carnivore diet concept is essentially an appeal to go back to our origins, both literally and symbolically. It serves as a reminder that we may achieve optimal health and vigor by adopting this ancient diet since our bodies are made to thrive on animal-based sustenance.

Individual encounters or reasons for researching the carnivorous diet

Examining the carnivore diet usually starts with a very personal experience or inspiration that pushes people to look for different ways to eat well and stay healthy. During this path, many people experience frustration, hardship, and an unwavering quest for health and vitality.

After years of suffering chronic health concerns that have resisted traditional treatment approaches, some people find solace in the carnivore diet. They are tired of depending on drugs to treat their autoimmune diseases (like rheumatoid arthritis) or digestive disorders (like irritable bowel syndrome) since they don't address the underlying source of their problems. Finally, desperate and with few other alternatives, they turn to the carnivore diet, which is a drastic break from conventional nutritional guidance and promises recovery and healing.

Some are driven by a desire to take back control of their body composition and weight. They've struggled for years with calorie tracking, yo-yo diets, and never-ending workout plans, and they're worn out and frustrated by the lack of long-lasting benefits. They're looking for a less complicated, more efficient way to control their weight—one that doesn't need starvation or repeated treadmill sessions. They consider the carnivore diet a means of overcoming a fixation with food and going back to eating in a way that is instinctive and natural.

Emotionally, deciding to research the carnivore diet is generally a combination of optimism and doubt. hope, since they've heard about the remarkable changes that those who follow a carnivorous diet have experienced. These include tales of weight loss, increased vitality, and recovery from chronic illnesses. Skepticism, since they are unsure of the diet's potential to benefit them and are aware of the debate and criticism surrounding it.

Above all, though, is a feeling of resolve—a readiness to question the status quo and defy expectations in the name of a better life. With little more than curiosity, bravery, and a firm conviction in the transformational power of food, people who are determined to improve their health and well-being set out on a carnivore diet adventure.

Individual problems, frustrations, and wants for health and vigor are deeply ingrained in the varied range of personal experiences and motives that have led people to investigate the carnivore diet. Whether motivated by a chronic disease, the desire for simplicity and independence, or weight control objectives, adopting a carnivore diet signifies a strong commitment to self-care and an openness to considering many routes to wellbeing.

Purpose of the book

This book's easy but profound goal is to give you the information, direction, and motivation you need to start your own trip with the carnivore diet and improve your health and well-being.

There is a lot of confusing nutrition advice and diet trends out there, but the carnivore diet stands out as being clear and easy to follow. Even though it's becoming more and more famous, a lot of people still don't know where to start or how to get around this different way of eating. That's why this book is useful.

My goal is to take the mystery out of the omnivore diet and give you all the information you need to get started, from knowing how the diet works in general to getting ideas for meals, shopping for food, and eating out. I have looked into the science behind the carnivore diet, looking at the research studies and data that support its possible benefits. I have also talked about some of the most common concerns and debates about it.

My other goal is to encourage you to take charge of your health and eat things that you feel good about. By giving you useful resources and tools like meal planning templates, food shopping lists, and tasty recipes that make the change easier and more enjoyable, we'll help you get through the tough parts of becoming a carnivore.

This book's goal is to give you the tools you need to get back your health, energy, and sense of well-being. We think that the foods you eat can change your life, whether you're trying to lose weight, deal with long-term health problems, or are just interested in a vegetarian diet. And with the advice and support given in these pages, we're confident that you can achieve the health and happiness you deserve.

Chapter 1: Understanding the Carnivore Diet

What is a carnivore diet?

Origins and development of the carnivore diet

Principles and rules of the carnivore diet

Different variations and approaches

What is a carnivore diet?

The carnivore diet is a dietary method that stresses the consumption of animal-based foods while excluding most plant-based foods. At its core, it's a radical departure from standard dietary rules that usually support a balanced intake of fruits, veggies, grains, and legumes. Instead, the carnivore diet argues for a diet mainly made of meat, fish, eggs, and certain dairy items.

At first glance, the carnivore diet may seem extreme or limiting. After all, it goes against the grain of what we've been told about the importance of eating a diverse array of foods to receive important nutrients. However, proponents of the carnivore diet say that humans developed as hunter-gatherers, depending on animal products as their main source of nutrition for millions of years. They think that our bodies are better suited to metabolize animal-based foods and that eating them entirely can lead to optimal health and energy.

The carnivore diet is often framed as a return to our primitive roots—a way of eating that matches the dietary habits of our ancestors. It's about simplifying our meals and reconnecting with the foods that supported us for ages before the rise of modern farms and processed foods. In essence, it's a rejection of the idea that we need a wide range of foods to be healthy and an acceptance of the power of animal-based nutrition to provide everything our bodies need to survive.

While the carnivore diet may seem easy in general— just eat meat, right?—there's actually quite a bit of complexity to it. There are different versions of the diet, ranging from strict carnivory, which removes all plant-based foods, to more flexible methods that allow for limited consumption of certain plant foods. Additionally, there's a wide range of animal-based foods to choose from, including beef, pork, chicken, fish, and eggs, as well as organ meats and dairy products.

The carnivore diet is also highly personal, meaning that what works for one person may not work for another. Some people thrive on a strict carnivore diet, experiencing profound changes in energy, mental clarity, and general health. Others may find that they need to add small amounts of plant-based foods or try different types of animal products to achieve optimal results.

The carnivore diet is about listening to your body and honoring its unique wants and tastes. It's a way of eating that promotes simplicity, sustainability, and the natural wisdom of our bodies. And while it may not be for everyone, for those who accept it, the carnivore diet can be a strong tool for reclaiming their health and energy.

Origins and development of the carnivore diet

The roots and development of the carnivore diet trace back to our oldest human ancestors, who subsisted mainly on animal-based foods as hunter-gatherers. For millions of years, before the rise of agriculture and modern food systems, humans walked the Earth as nomadic hunters, depending on their skills to find and gather food from the natural environment.

Our ancestors' diet consisted mainly of meat, fish, eggs, and certain animal-derived goods like bone marrow and organ meats. These foods provide the necessary nutrients needed for life, including protein, fat, vitamins, and minerals. In this ancestral diet, there was little to no dependence on plant-based foods, as agriculture had not yet been created and fruits, veggies, grains, and legumes were not easily available year-round.

The move to agriculture marked a major shift in human dietary habits, as people began to grow and domesticate plants for food. Over time, grains like wheat, rice, and corn became staple crops in many countries, and plant-based foods came to rule the human diet. However, it's important to note that while agriculture brought about major advancements in food production and human civilization, it also introduced dietary changes that some say may not have been ideal for human health.

Fast forward to the modern age, and we find ourselves grappling with a myriad of health problems that were nearly nonexistent in our hunter-gatherer ancestors. Chronic diseases like obesity, diabetes, heart disease, and autoimmune conditions are on the rise, despite improvements in medical technology and healthcare.

In reaction to these health issues, a greater number of people are looking to ancestral dietary approaches like the carnivore diet as a way to reclaim their health and energy. The carnivore diet represents a return to our primitive roots – a way of eating that closely matches the food habits of our hunter-gatherer ancestors. By focusing on animal-based foods while excluding most plant-based foods, proponents of the carnivore diet believe that it's possible to optimize health, improve energy levels, and treat a variety of health problems.

The evolution of the carnivore diet is also affected by current scientific studies, which have shed light on the possible health benefits of animal-based nutrition. Studies have shown that animal products are rich sources of important nutrients like protein, omega-3 fatty acids, vitamins, and minerals, which are crucial for supporting general health and well-being. Additionally, research on low-carbohydrate and ketogenic diets has given further evidence for the idea that reducing carbohydrate intake and increasing fat and protein consumption may have metabolic and health benefits.

The roots and development of the carnivore diet are deeply rooted in our ancestral past and shaped by current scientific knowledge of nutrition and health. By adopting a dietary approach that values animal-based foods while excluding most plant-based foods, proponents of the carnivore diet believe that it's possible to reclaim our health and energy in a world that seems increasingly at odds with our evolutionary history.

Principles and rules of the carnivore diet

The carnivore diet is based on several key concepts and rules that guide its application and practice. At its core, the omnivore diet is a simple yet strict dietary approach that promotes the consumption of animal-based foods while excluding most plant-based foods. Here are the basic ideas and rules of the carnivore diet:

Emphasis on Animal-Based Foods: The main focus of the carnivore diet is on eating animal-based foods such as meat, fish, poultry, eggs, and certain dairy products. These foods provide important nutrients like protein, fat, vitamins, and minerals that are necessary for good health and well-being.
absence of plant-based foods: One of the main features of the carnivore diet is the absence of most plant-based foods, including fruits, veggies, grains, legumes, nuts, seeds, and processed foods made from plants. The reasoning behind this restriction is that plant-based foods may contain anti-nutrients,

toxins, and other substances that could possibly harm the body or contribute to health problems.

Focus on Whole Foods: The carnivore diet emphasizes the consumption of whole, slightly processed animal-based foods over processed or refined goods. This includes picking fresh or frozen meats, wild-caught fish, pasture-raised poultry, and organic eggs whenever possible, while avoiding processed meats, salted meats, and other highly processed animal products.

Hydration: While water is not exactly a part of the carnivore diet, it's important to stay hydrated by drinking an adequate amount of water throughout the day. Some carnivore diet followers also include bone broth as a source of water and extra nutrients.

Optional Supplements: While the carnivore diet aims to provide all necessary nutrients through animal-based foods, some people may choose to supplement with certain vitamins or minerals to ensure nutritional balance. Common nutrients on the carnivore diet include vitamin D, omega-3 fatty acids, and electrolytes like salt, potassium, and magnesium.

Listen to Your Body: As with any dietary plan, it's important to listen to your body's hunger cues, energy levels, and general well-being while following the carnivore diet. Some people may find that they thrive on a strict carnivore diet, while others may need to try different variations or include small amounts of plant-based foods to meet their nutritional needs and tastes.

The principles and rules of the carnivore diet focus on favoring nutrient-dense animal-based foods while excluding most plant-based foods. By adhering to these principles and listening to their bodies, people can experience the possible health benefits of the carnivore diet while supporting their general health and well-being.

Different variations and approaches

The carnivore diet may seem straightforward at first glance – just eat meat, right? However, there are actually several different variations and approaches to this dietary lifestyle, each with its own nuances and guidelines. From strict carnivory to more flexible approaches that incorporate small amounts of plant-based foods, the carnivore diet offers options to suit a variety of preferences and dietary needs.

Strict Carnivore Diet: The strict carnivore diet, also known as zero-carb or all-meat diet, is the most extreme version of the carnivore diet. Followers of this approach consume only animal-based foods and exclude all plant-based foods entirely. This includes meat, fish, poultry, eggs, and certain dairy products like butter and cheese. The strict carnivore diet is based on the belief that humans evolved as obligate carnivores and that plant-based foods are unnecessary or even harmful for optimal health.

Animal-Based Carnivore Diet: This variation of the carnivore diet allows for the inclusion of certain animal-derived products that may not strictly fit into the category of meat, fish, or eggs. This can include foods like bone broth, collagen supplements, and gelatin, which are derived from animal bones, connective tissues, and skin. While these foods are not technically meat, they are considered acceptable on the animal-based carnivore diet due to their nutrient density and potential health benefits.

Dairy-Inclusive Carnivore Diet: Some individuals on the carnivore diet choose to include certain dairy products like butter, cheese, and heavy cream. While dairy is technically derived from animal sources, it can be controversial within the carnivore community due to concerns about lactose intolerance, casein sensitivity, and other potential issues. However, for those who tolerate dairy well and enjoy its taste and versatility, incorporating dairy products into the carnivore diet can provide additional variety and flavor.

Nose-to-Tail Carnivore Diet: This approach to the carnivore diet emphasizes the consumption of the whole animal, including organ meats, bones, and other less commonly consumed parts. Organ meats like liver, kidney, and heart are particularly nutrient-dense and provide essential vitamins and minerals that may be lacking in muscle meat alone. Additionally, bone broth, marrow, and cartilage are rich sources of collagen, gelatin, and other beneficial compounds that support joint health, gut health, and overall well-being.

Carnivore Diet with Limited Plant Foods: While the carnivore diet typically excludes most plant-based foods, some individuals may choose to incorporate small amounts of certain plant foods for variety or personal preference. This can include non-sweet fruits like avocado, olives, and coconut, as well as low-carbohydrate vegetables like leafy greens, cruciferous vegetables, and squash. While these foods are technically allowed on the carnivore diet, they are consumed sparingly and in small quantities to maintain the focus on animal-based nutrition.

Cyclic Carnivore Diet: This approach involves cycling periods of strict carnivory with periods of more flexible eating that may include small amounts of plant-based foods or occasional indulgences. For example, someone following a cyclic carnivore diet may adhere strictly to animal-based foods during the week and then enjoy a meal or two with friends or family that includes non-carnivore foods on the weekends. This allows for greater dietary flexibility while still reaping the potential benefits of the carnivore diet.

The variations and approaches to the carnivore diet offer flexibility and customization to suit individual preferences, dietary needs, and health goals. Whether following a strict carnivore diet or incorporating small amounts of plant-based foods, the key is to prioritize nutrient-dense animal-based nutrition while listening to your body and making choices that support your overall health and well-being.

Chapter 2: Chapter 2: The Science Behind the Carnivore Diet

Nutritional makeup of animal products

Debunking popular myths and misunderstandings

Research studies and evidence supporting the carnivore diet

Potential benefits and drawbacks

Nutritional makeup of animal products

The nutritional makeup of animal products is varied and highly valuable, providing important nutrients that are crucial for maintaining excellent health and well-being. Meat, fish, chicken, eggs, and dairy products are rich sources of protein, fat, vitamins, and minerals, making them vital components of a balanced and nutritious diet.

Protein: Animal products are prized for their high-quality protein content, which is necessary for building and healing tissues, supporting muscle growth and maintenance, and maintaining general body function. Proteins found in animal products contain all the necessary amino acids that the body cannot make on its own, making them full sources of protein that are easily absorbed and utilized by the body.

Fat: Animal goods are also rich in healthy fats, including saturated fats, monounsaturated fats, and omega-3 fatty acids. While saturated fats have been demonized in the past, new research shows that they play a key role in hormone production, brain function, and cellular integrity. Monounsaturated fats, found in foods like fatty fish and chicken, have been linked to heart health and may help lower cholesterol levels. Omega-3 fatty acids, abundant in fatty fish like salmon and mackerel, are important for brain function, heart health, and lowering inflammation in the body.

Vitamins: Animal products are great sources of several important vitamins, including vitamin B12, vitamin D, vitamin A, and vitamin K2. Vitamin B12, found mainly in meat, chicken, fish, and dairy products, is necessary for nerve function, DNA synthesis, and the formation of red blood cells. Vitamin D, mainly obtained from fatty fish and egg yolks, is important for bone health, immune function, and mood regulation. Vitamin A, found in the liver, eggs, and dairy products, is important for eyes, immune function, and skin health. Vitamin K2, found in fermented dairy products and certain animal fats, plays a key role in bone metabolism and cardiovascular health.

Minerals: Animal goods are abundant sources of important minerals like iron, zinc, selenium, and calcium. Iron, found in red meat, chicken, and fish, is necessary for oxygen transport, energy production, and immune function. Zinc, found in meat, shrimp, and dairy products, is important for immune function, wound healing, and sexual health. Selenium, found in seafood, meat, and eggs, works as a strong antioxidant and supports thyroid function. Calcium, found in dairy products like milk, cheese, and yogurt, is important for bone health, muscle function, and nerve communication.

Animal goods are nutrient-dense foods that provide a wide range of important nutrients, including protein, fat, vitamins, and minerals. Incorporating a range of animal products into your diet can help ensure that you meet your nutritional needs and support your general health and well-being.

Debunking common myths and misconceptions about the carnivore diet is important to provide accurate information and help people make informed decisions about their dietary choices. While the carnivore diet has gained popularity in recent years, it's also been surrounded by a fair share of criticism and misunderstanding. Here, we'll cover some of the most popular myths and misconceptions about the carnivore diet:

Myth: The carnivore diet lacks important nutrients. One of the most common misunderstandings about the carnivore diet is that it's nutritionally deficient and lacks essential nutrients. However, animal-based foods like meat, fish, poultry, and eggs are rich sources of protein, fat, vitamins, and minerals, giving all the necessary nutrients it needs to grow. With proper planning and a range of food choices, followers of the carnivore diet can meet their nutritional goals without counting on plant-based foods.

Myth: The carnivore diet is dangerous and unsustainable: Another misunderstanding is that the carnivore diet is unhealthy and unstable in the long run. While the carnivore diet may seem extreme to some, there is growing evidence to suggest that it can be a safe and effective dietary method for certain people. Many people report improvements in weight control, energy levels, digestive health, and general well-being after following the carnivore diet.

Myth: The carnivore diet causes nutrient deficiencies: Some people worry that eliminating plant-based foods from the diet will lead to nutrient deficiencies, especially in vitamins and minerals found in fruits and veggies. However, animal-based foods are nutrient-dense and provide all the necessary nutrients the body needs to work optimally. Additionally, many users of the carnivore diet report changes in nutrient intake and usage due to reduced inflammation and better gut health.

Myth: The carnivore diet increases the chance of heart disease: There's a common misunderstanding that the high fat content of animal-based foods in the carnivore diet increases the risk of heart disease and other cardiovascular problems. However, new research shows that saturated fats from animal sources may not be as dangerous as once thought and may even have positive effects on heart health when eaten as part of a healthy diet. Additionally, many followers of the carnivore diet report changes in cholesterol readings and other signs of heart health.

Myth: The carnivore diet is only for weight loss: While some people may follow the carnivore diet for weight loss, it's not the main goal or benefit of this dietary method. Many people choose the carnivore diet for reasons beyond weight management, including better digestive health, reducing inflammation, increasing energy levels, and treating chronic health conditions.

Research studies and evidence supporting the carnivore diet

Research studies and evidence supporting the carnivore diet are continually evolving, shedding light on the potential benefits and implications of this dietary approach. While the carnivore diet is still relatively understudied compared to more conventional dietary patterns, there is a growing body of research that suggests it may have potential health benefits for certain individuals. Here, we'll explore some of the key research studies and evidence supporting the carnivore diet:

Improvements in Metabolic Health: Several studies have found that the carnivore diet may lead to improvements in metabolic health markers such as blood sugar levels, insulin sensitivity, and lipid profiles. For example, a study published in the Journal of Medical Case Reports documented significant improvements in blood sugar control and insulin sensitivity in a patient with type 2 diabetes following a strict carnivore diet for six months. Additionally, research has shown that the carnivore diet can lead to reductions in markers of inflammation and oxidative stress, which are implicated in the development of metabolic diseases like diabetes and heart disease.

Weight Loss and Body Composition: Some research suggests that the carnivore diet may be effective for weight loss and improving body composition. A study published in the American Journal of Clinical Nutrition found that a high-protein, low-carbohydrate diet – similar to the carnivore diet – resulted in greater weight loss and fat loss compared to a standard low-fat diet. Other studies have reported similar findings, with participants experiencing significant reductions in body weight, body fat percentage, and waist circumference after following a carnivore or low-carb diet.

Gut Health and Digestive Function: Emerging research suggests that the carnivore diet may have positive effects on gut health and digestive function. A study published in the journal Gut Microbes found that a meat-based diet led to favorable changes in gut microbiota composition, including increases in beneficial bacteria and reductions in pathogenic bacteria. Additionally, many individuals report improvements in digestive symptoms such as bloating, gas, and abdominal discomfort after adopting the carnivore diet, suggesting that it may be beneficial for those with gastrointestinal issues.

Autoimmune Conditions and Inflammatory Diseases: Preliminary evidence suggests that the carnivore diet may be helpful for managing autoimmune conditions and inflammatory diseases. Case studies and anecdotal reports have documented improvements in symptoms of conditions like rheumatoid arthritis, psoriasis, and inflammatory bowel disease after adopting a carnivore or low-carb, high-fat diet. While more research is needed to understand the mechanisms underlying these effects, the anti-inflammatory and immune-modulating properties of animal-based foods may play a role.

Mental Health and Cognitive Function: Some research suggests that the carnivore diet may have positive effects on mental health and cognitive function. A study published in the journal Nutritional Neuroscience found that a high-protein, low-carbohydrate diet improved mood, cognitive function, and overall well-being in overweight and obese individuals. Other studies have reported similar findings, with participants experiencing improvements in mood, focus, and mental clarity after following a carnivore or low-carb diet.

While the research supporting the carnivore diet is promising, it's important to note that much of the evidence is still preliminary and more research is needed to fully understand its long-term effects and implications. Additionally, the carnivore diet may not be suitable for everyone and individual responses to the diet can vary. As with any dietary approach, it's essential to consult with a healthcare professional before making significant changes to your diet, especially if you have underlying health conditions or concerns.

Potential benefits and drawbacks

The carnivore diet, like any dietary plan, comes with its own set of possible benefits and downsides. While some people may experience major gains in health and well-being on the carnivore diet, others may face difficulties or harmful effects. Here, we'll discuss some of the possible benefits and downsides of the carnivore diet:

Potential Benefits:

Weight Loss: One of the most frequently stated benefits of the carnivore diet is weight loss. By removing carbohydrates and focusing on protein and fat-rich animal foods, many people find that they naturally consume fewer calories and experience reductions in body weight and body fat percentage.

Improved Metabolic Health: Research shows that the carnivore diet may lead to changes in metabolic health factors such as blood sugar levels, insulin sensitivity, and lipid profiles. Some studies have found decreases in fasting blood glucose, insulin levels, and markers of inflammation after following a carnivore or low-carbohydrate diet.

Reduced Inflammation: The carnivore diet is naturally low in anti-nutrients and possible inflammatory triggers found in plant-based foods. Many people report decreases in signs of inflammation-related conditions such as arthritis, autoimmune diseases, and digestive problems after following the carnivore diet.

Simplified Eating: The carnivore diet gives a simple and easy approach to eating, with no need to count calories, track macronutrients, or plan complex meals. For some people, this ease can be freeing and help reduce stress and anxiety around food.

Increased Energy and Mental Clarity: Many fans of the carnivore diet claim changes in energy levels, mental clarity, and brain function. By stabilizing blood sugar levels and offering a steady source of fuel from fat and protein, the carnivore diet may support prolonged energy and attention throughout the day.

Potential Drawbacks:

Nutritional Deficiencies: One of the main concerns with the carnivore diet is the possibility of nutritional deficiencies, especially in vitamins, minerals, and fiber. Since the diet excludes most plant-based foods, followers may be at risk of poor intake of nutrients like vitamin C, vitamin K, potassium, and fiber, which are usually found in fruits, veggies, and grains.

Gut Health Issues: While some people experience changes in digestive health on the carnivore diet, others may face problems such as constipation, diarrhea, or disruptions in gut bacteria makeup. The lack of dietary fiber and prebiotic substances found in plant-based foods can impact bowel movements and gut health for some people.

Challenges with Socialization and Convenience: Following a carnivore diet may present challenges when dining out, visiting social events, or traveling, where plant-based choices are more easily available. Additionally, finding high-quality animal products can be expensive or inconvenient for some people, depending on their location and income.

Potential Long-Term Health Risks: While short-term studies have shown the potential benefits of the carnivore diet, the long-term health effects are still unknown. Some experts voice worry about the possible risks of eating large amounts of red meat and saturated fat over time, including a higher risk of heart disease, certain cancers, and other chronic health conditions.

Individual Variability: The carnivore diet may not be good for everyone, and individual reactions can vary greatly. While some people thrive on a strict carnivore diet, others may experience adverse effects such as tiredness, vitamin deficits, or digestive problems. It's important to listen to your body and make changes as needed to ensure the diet is sustainable and supportive of your general health and well-being.

In conclusion, the carnivore diet offers possible benefits such as weight loss, better metabolic health, reduced inflammation, and increased energy and mental focus. However, it also comes with possible downsides such as nutritional deficits, gut health issues, challenges with socialization and ease, potential long-term health risks, and individual variability. As with any food approach, it's important to weigh the possible benefits and downsides and make informed choices based on your individual needs, tastes, and health goals. Consulting with a healthcare professional or qualified dietitian can also provide useful advice and support in handling the carnivore diet safely and successfully.

Chapter 3: Getting Started on the Carnivore Diet

Getting ready for the change

Foods to eat and stay away from

Advice on grocery shopping and meal planning

Common challenges and how to overcome them

Getting ready for the change

To guarantee a seamless and effective adjustment, meticulous planning, thoughtful analysis, and awareness are necessary while preparing for the shift to a carnivorous diet. It might assist in setting you up for success to take the time to prepare yourself both psychologically and practically, whether you are new to the carnivorous lifestyle or are switching from another nutritional strategy. When getting ready to make the switch to a carnivorous diet, keep the following important steps in mind:

Inform Yourself: Invest some time in familiarizing yourself with the tenets and standards of the carnivore diet before implementing any major dietary adjustments. Learn about the kinds of foods that are permitted on the diet, along with any possible advantages and disadvantages. Knowing the science behind the carnivore diet will empower you to make wise choices and establish reasonable expectations for the change.

Establish Specific Objectives: Analyze your motivations for wanting to switch to a carnivorous diet and make sure your goals are specific and doable. Whether your goal is to become healthier, reduce weight, or deal with a particular health concern, having a distinct purpose can help you stay motivated and concentrated during the change.

Gradual Transition: Rather than making drastic changes all at once, think about introducing the carnivorous diet gradually. Start by progressively cutting back on your carbohydrate intake and gradually increasing your intake of meals derived from animals. By going slowly, you can reduce the possibility of negative impacts and make the change easier to handle.

Stock Up on Essentials: Give yourself enough time to prepare the meals and products you'll need to sustain your new, carnivorous diet before beginning the diet. Give special attention to nutrient-dense, high-quality animal products, including dairy, fish, poultry, eggs, and meat. To optimize nutritional quality, try to find products that are pasture-raised and grass-fed wherever feasible.

Meal Planning and Preparation: To facilitate your shift to a carnivorous diet, make a plan for your meals and start cooking them ahead of time. To make meals exciting and fun, try out various recipes and cooking techniques. If you want to prepare meals more quickly and easily, think about investing in kitchen appliances and other types of equipment.

Hydration and Electrolytes: When switching to a carnivorous diet, be mindful of your electrolyte and hydration levels. Due to the low carbohydrate content of the diet, your body may initially excrete more water and electrolytes, which might result in electrolyte imbalances and dehydration. To maintain hydration and general well-being, be sure you drink lots of water and think about taking an electrolyte supplement as necessary.

Pay attention to your body. Lastly, pay attention to your body throughout this transition period and modify your strategy based on your feelings. Be mindful of your body's signals about appetite, energy, digestion, and general health, and modify as necessary. Always keep in mind that every person's experience with the carnivorous diet is different, so you really need to figure out what suits you the most.

foods to eat and stay away from

Success in implementing a carnivore diet depends on knowing which items to include and which to avoid. You may maintain your health and well-being on a carnivore diet by emphasizing nutrient-dense animal-based meals and eliminating some plant-based items. Below is a summary of foods to consume and stay away from:

Foods to try:

Meat: The main component of a carnivorous diet, meat ought to be the main attraction at mealtimes. Try to consume a range of meats, such as game, venison, lamb, hog, and beef. When feasible, opt for fatty slices because they are high in nutrients and help you feel full.

Fish and Seafood: Rich in protein, omega-3 fatty acids, and vital vitamins and minerals, fish and seafood are great meal choices. Add a range of shellfish, such as shrimp, crab, and oysters, and fatty fish, such as salmon, mackerel, sardines, and herring.

Poultry: A carnivore diet can also contain poultry, such as duck, turkey, and chicken. For the best taste and nutritional value, choose dark meat slices that still have their skin on. For added nutrition, think about consuming organ meats like liver, heart, and gizzards.

Eggs: A nutrient-dense meal that fits well into a carnivorous diet is eggs. For eggs with greater nutritional content, wherever feasible, choose pasture-raised or omega-3-fortified eggs. There are several ways to prepare eggs, such as boiling, poaching, frying, and scrambling.

Dairy Products: Some people decide to include cheese, butter, ghee, heavy cream, and other dairy products in their carnivorous diet. To optimize nutritional advantages, choose premium, full-fat dairy products from cows grown on pasture.

Bone Broth: Suitable for a carnivorous diet, bone broth is a refreshing and nutritious drink. It's a great supplement to your diet because it's full of minerals, collagen, gelatin, and amino acids. For maximum nutritional value, try using bones from animals grown on pasture or on grass when creating homemade bone broth.

Foods to stay away from:

Plant-Based Foods: The majority of plant-based foods, such as fruits, vegetables, grains, legumes, nuts, seeds, and processed foods made from plants, are not allowed in a carnivorous diet. These meals tend to be heavy in anti-nutrients, carbs, and other substances that might be hard to digest or could obstruct the absorption of nutrients.

Processed Meats: Although fresh, unprocessed meats are an essential part of a carnivore's diet, processed meats such as bacon, sausages, jerky, and deli meats are to be avoided or used in moderation. These goods frequently include preservatives, added sugars, and other ingredients that might not be in line with the carnivore diet's tenets.

Vegetable and Seed Oils: On a carnivorous diet, it is best to stay away from vegetable and seed oils such as sunflower, canola, maize, and soybean oils. Due to their high content of inflammatory omega-6 fatty acids, these oils may put the body at risk for oxidative stress and inflammation.

Processed and Packaged Foods: On a carnivore diet, processed and packaged foods—such as snacks, candies, chips, and other convenience foods—should be avoided. These goods frequently include large amounts of added sugars, bad fats, carbs, and artificial additives, all of which can be harmful to one's health.

Sugary Drinks: On a carnivorous diet, sugary drinks, including soda, fruit juice, sports drinks, and sweetened teas, should be avoided. Due to their high sugar content and lack of nutritional value, these drinks might cause weight gain, insulin resistance, and other health problems.

Alcohol: Because alcohol contains carbs and may disrupt ketosis and fat metabolism, it is not allowed on the carnivorous diet. Alcohol use may also worsen judgment, interfere, with sleep, and increase the risk of dehydration.

Advice on grocery shopping and meal planning

Planning meals and doing your grocery shopping are crucial to following the carnivore diet successfully. You can make sure you have all you need to maintain your health and well-being on this dietary strategy by carefully organizing your meals and choosing premium animal-based items. Here are some pointers for grocery shopping and meal planning while following a carnivorous diet:

Make a Weekly Meal Plan: Set aside some time each week to organize your meals for the following days. Think about the kinds of meats, fish, poultry, eggs, and dairy products you want to use in your dishes. You should also think about any other flavors or ingredients you might require. You can maintain organization and make sure you have everything you need on hand by creating a meal plan.

Emphasis on foods rich in nutrients: Animal-based foods that are high in nutrients and include important vitamins, minerals, and macronutrients should be given priority for meal planning. Select a range of meats, such as game, deer, lamb, cattle, and hog, and fatty fish like sardines, mackerel, and salmon. For added nutrition, incorporate organ meats such as the liver, heart, and kidney. You may also add eggs and dairy products to your diet as needed.

Think about batch cooking: on a carnivorous diet, this may be a time-saving method for preparing meals. Think of preparing big quantities of meat, fish, or fowl at once and dividing them up for several meals over the week. Additionally, you may make more bone broth and freeze it in portion-free freezer bags for convenient access.

Add Some Easy Side Dishes: Although animal-based foods are the main emphasis of the carnivore diet, you can still improve your meals by adding some easy side dishes or sauces. To add taste and diversity to your meals, think about including ingredients like salt, pepper, herbs, spices, and animal fats like butter, ghee, or tallow.

Purchase High-Quality Ingredients: Whenever feasible, give top priority to premium animal products that have been grown on pasture or grass when grocery shopping for a carnivorous diet. Seek out poultry, fish, and meats that have not been treated with hormones, antibiotics, or other contaminants. For the most nutritious value, select dairy products from grass-fed cows and eggs from birds kept on pasture.

See the farmer's markets and butchers in your area: For the carnivore diet, high-quality animal-based items can be found in local farmers' markets and butchers. These places frequently have a more extensive assortment of seafood, poultry, and meats in addition to unique foods like organ meats and bone broth. Developing a rapport with nearby farmers can also assist in guaranteeing that you have access to the healthiest and freshest foods.
Pay close attention to the labels: When buying processed or packaged animal products, such as bacon, sausages, or deli meats, be sure to carefully read the labels and select those that have few ingredients and don't include any

artificial additives, added sugars, or preservatives. Choose goods that have had the least amount of processing and are most like the original.

Stock Up on Staples: If you follow a carnivorous diet, keep your pantry well-stocked with basic foods like bone broth, salt, pepper, herbs, and spices. Keeping these supplies on hand will allow you to create meals quickly and simply without needing to make frequent visits to the grocery store.

Think About Frozen Choices: When it comes to meal planning and grocery shopping for a carnivorous diet, frozen meats, fish, and poultry might be practical choices. Because frozen meals can be kept for extended periods of time and are frequently just as healthy as fresh ones, they help cut down on waste and guarantee that you always have food on hand.

Be Adaptable and Try New Things: Lastly, don't be scared to be adaptable and try out various carnivore diet foods and recipes. To keep your meals interesting and pleasurable, experiment with different cooking techniques, new meat cuts, and flavorings and seasonings. Pay attention to your body's signals of hunger and desire, and modify your grocery list and meal plan as necessary.

You may position yourself for success and make sure you have all you need to support your health and well-being on this dietary strategy by paying attention to these guidelines for meal planning and grocery shopping on the carnivore diet. Eating a carnivorous diet may be enjoyable and healthful if you plan ahead, use excellent foods, and are ready to try new things.

Common challenges and how to overcome them

Embarking on a carnivore diet can be a transformative journey towards improved health and well-being. However, like any significant lifestyle change, it comes with its own set of challenges. Understanding these challenges and knowing how to overcome them can help you navigate the carnivore diet successfully and achieve your health goals. Here are some common challenges and strategies for overcoming them:

Carbohydrate Withdrawal Symptoms: One of the most common challenges when transitioning to a carnivore diet is experiencing withdrawal symptoms from carbohydrates. As your body adjusts to the absence of carbohydrates, you may experience symptoms such as headaches, fatigue, irritability, and cravings. To overcome carbohydrate withdrawal symptoms, stay hydrated, prioritize electrolyte balance, and gradually reduce your carbohydrate intake rather than making abrupt changes. Consuming plenty of water, electrolytes, and nutrient-dense animal-based foods can help alleviate symptoms and support your transition to a carnivore diet.

Social Pressure and Judgement: Another challenge of the carnivore diet is navigating social situations and dealing with pressure or judgment from others. Friends, family members, and colleagues may question or criticize your dietary choices, leading to feelings of isolation or frustration. To overcome social pressure, communicate openly with others about your reasons for following the carnivore diet and educate them about its potential benefits. Focus on your own health and well-being rather than seeking validation from others, and surround yourself with supportive individuals who respect your dietary choices.

Digestive Issues: Some individuals may experience digestive issues when transitioning to the carnivore diet, such as bloating, gas, constipation, or diarrhea. These issues may arise due to changes in gut microbiota composition, alterations in bile production, or differences in nutrient absorption. To overcome digestive issues, start slowly and gradually increasing your intake of animal-based foods over time. Incorporate bone broth, fermented foods, and digestive enzymes to support gut health and digestion. Pay attention to how different foods and cooking methods affect your digestion, and adjust your diet accordingly.

Nutrient Deficiencies: While animal-based foods are nutrient-dense, some individuals may still be at risk of nutrient deficiencies on the carnivore diet, particularly if they restrict their food choices or have underlying health issues. Common nutrient deficiencies in the carnivore diet include vitamin C, vitamin K, potassium, and fiber. To overcome nutrient deficiencies, prioritize a variety of animal-based foods, including different cuts of meat, fatty fish, organ meats, eggs, and dairy products. Consider incorporating small amounts of nutrient-rich plant-based foods like liver, and bone marrow, and small amounts of low-carbohydrate vegetables to ensure you're meeting your nutritional needs.

Meal Planning and Variety: Another challenge of the carnivore diet is meal planning and maintaining variety in your diet. Eating the same foods day after day can lead to boredom, food fatigue, and nutrient imbalances. To overcome this challenge, experiment with different cuts of meat, cooking methods, and seasonings to keep your meals interesting and enjoyable. Incorporate a variety of meats, fish, poultry, eggs, and dairy products into your diet to ensure you're getting a wide range of nutrients. Consider trying new recipes, joining online communities or forums for recipe ideas and inspiration, and meal prepping to save time and effort.

Cravings and Emotional Eating: Cravings for carbohydrates or non-carnivore foods can be a significant challenge when following the carnivore diet, particularly during times of stress or emotional upheaval. To overcome cravings and emotional eating, focus on nutrient-dense animal-based foods that provide satiety and satisfaction. Practice mindfulness and self-awareness around food choices, and find alternative ways to cope with stress or emotions, such as exercise, meditation, or hobbies. Identify triggers for cravings and develop strategies to address them, such as keeping tempting foods out of the house or finding healthier alternatives.

Budget Constraints: Following the carnivore diet can be expensive, especially if you prioritize high-quality, pasture-raised, and grass-fed animal products. Budget constraints may limit your ability to purchase these premium products, which can be a significant challenge for some individuals. To overcome budget constraints, prioritize the most affordable animal-based foods available in your area, such as ground beef, chicken thighs, and canned fish. Consider buying in bulk, purchasing cheaper cuts of meat, and taking advantage of sales, discounts, and coupons to save money. Explore alternative sources of protein, such as eggs, dairy products, and organ meats, which tend to be more affordable than premium cuts of meat.

Adherence and Long-Term Sustainability: Finally, one of the biggest challenges of the carnivore diet is adherence and long-term sustainability. While many individuals experience initial success and improvements in health on the carnivore diet, maintaining this dietary approach over the long term can be challenging for some. To overcome this challenge, focus on flexibility, balance, and moderation in your dietary choices. Listen to your body's hunger cues and cravings, and allow yourself occasional indulgences or deviations from the strict carnivore diet when appropriate. Remember that the carnivore diet is not one-size-fits-all, and it's okay to make adjustments to suit your individual needs and preferences.

The carnivore diet presents several common challenges that individuals may encounter when transitioning to this dietary approach. By understanding these challenges and implementing strategies to overcome them, you can navigate the carnivore diet successfully and achieve your health goals. Remember to prioritize nutrient-dense animal-based foods, practice mindfulness and self-awareness around food choices, and seek support from healthcare professionals or online communities if needed. With dedication, perseverance, and a willingness to adapt, you can overcome challenges and thrive

Loss of weight and changes to body composition

increased vitality and clarity of thought

Handling long-term illnesses and ailments

Improvements in digestive system and gut health

Hormonal equilibrium and metabolic well-being

Loss of weight and changes to body composition

Many people who start a carnivore diet have the common objective of losing weight and changing their body composition. Although the carnivore diet focuses primarily on general health and well-being, many people find that following this eating strategy significantly improves their ability to control their weight and body composition. Here, we'll look at the ways in which the carnivore diet can help with weight reduction and body composition modifications, as well as the variables that influence these results:

Decreased Calorie Intake: A lower calorie intake is one of the key causes of weight loss in those following a carnivorous diet. Naturally abundant in protein and fat, animal-based meals like meat, fish, and poultry can help regulate appetite and reduce overall food consumption since they are extremely satiating. Furthermore, removing processed foods and carbs from the diet can help cut calories even further, resulting in a calorie deficit and weight reduction.

Enhanced Satiety and Fullness: Foods high in fat and protein from animals are known to increase feelings of satiety and fullness, which can help cut down on overindulging and between-meal snacking. Those following a carnivore diet may naturally eat fewer calories without feeling restricted or hungry, which can result in weight loss and improvements in body composition. Nutrient-dense animal products should be prioritized, while processed foods and carbs should be avoided.

Enhanced Fat Burning: The carnivore diet encourages ketosis, a state in which the body predominantly burns fat rather of carbs for energy. Those following a carnivorous diet can enhance fat burning and aid in weight reduction by limiting their intake of carbohydrates and boosting their consumption of fat, especially if they have metabolic problems or are insulin resistant. Additionally, ketosis suppresses hunger, which helps with weight reduction and changes in body composition.

Preservation of Lean Muscle Mass: The carnivore diet places a strong emphasis on meals high in protein from animals, which are crucial for maintaining lean muscle mass. This is in contrast to many fad diets that encourage drastic calorie restriction and muscle loss in order to achieve quick weight reduction. Sufficient consumption of protein is essential for preserving muscle mass while losing weight and fostering a normal metabolism. Those following a carnivorous diet can enhance their body composition and boost muscle retention by emphasizing resistance exercise and protein.

Diminished Water Weight: The body stores carbohydrates as glycogen, which attaches itself to water molecules. Glycogen reserves are depleted during the carnivore diet's restriction of carbs, which causes a fast loss of water weight in the early phases of the diet. Even though the first weight reduction may be mostly the result of fluid changes rather than fat loss, it can nevertheless improve body composition and encourage people to stick to the diet.

Enhancements in Metabolic Well-Being: It has been demonstrated that the carnivore diet enhances lipid profiles, insulin sensitivity, and blood sugar levels as indicators of metabolic health. The carnivore diet reduces inflammation, stabilizes blood sugar, and encourages fat burning to help treat underlying metabolic problems that lead to obesity and weight gain. Weight reduction and changes in body composition that are more long-term and sustainable may result from these metabolic improvements.

Individual Variability: It's crucial to remember that each person will experience weight reduction and changes in body composition while following a carnivorous diet differently. Individual results can be influenced by a variety of factors, including age, gender, heredity, metabolic rate, exercise level, and diet adherence. While some people may lose weight quickly and dramatically, others may lose weight more gradually over time. Furthermore, any dietary strategy, including the carnivore diet, will always have oscillations and plateaus in weight reduction; they should be accepted as normal parts of the process.

The carnivore diet's concentration on nutrient-dense animal-based meals, decreased calorie intake, enhanced satiety, fat adaptation, and metabolic improvements often result in weight reduction and changes in body composition. A person following the carnivore diet can accomplish long-term weight reduction and improvements in body composition by emphasizing meals high in protein and fat, reducing their intake of carbs and processed foods, and concentrating on their general health and well-being. However, since individual outcomes may vary and improvement may take time, it's essential to approach weight reduction with patience, consistency, and a long-term view. Speaking with a medical expert or certified dietitian can also offer tailored advice and assistance in reaching your body composition and weight reduction objectives while following a carnivorous diet.

Increased vitality and clarity of thought

Enhanced vitality and well-being are mostly dependent on improved energy and mental clarity. People who possess strong levels of energy and mental clarity are better able to take on daily responsibilities, exercise, and stay focused and productive all day long. It takes a comprehensive strategy that addresses many facets of lifestyle, such as nutrition, exercise, sleep, stress management, and mental health, to achieve and maintain increased energy and mental clarity.

Diet High in Nutrients: Eating a diet high in nutrients is essential for promoting increased energy and mental clarity. The body gets its energy and building blocks from a balanced diet that includes macronutrients (protein, carbs, and fats) and micronutrients (vitamins and minerals). Whole grains, fruits, and vegetables are high in complex carbs, which release energy gradually. Lean proteins and healthy fats, on the other hand, aid in maintaining cognitive function and blood sugar stability.

Hydration: Sustaining energy levels and mental performance requires enough hydration. Fatigue, a loss of concentration, and compromised cognitive function can result from even slight dehydration. Throughout the day, drinking lots of water increases the body's ability to eliminate waste, carry nutrients, and stay hydrated. It also enhances general well-being. Try to consume eight glasses of water or more each day, and modify your amount according to your needs, the weather, and your degree of exercise.

Frequent Exercise: Getting regular exercise is a great method to increase energy and improve mental clarity. Exercise increases mood and cognitive performance, increases blood flow to the brain, and triggers the production of endorphins, or feel-good chemicals. Including a variety of aerobic, strength, and flexibility workouts in your regimen will help boost your mood, lower your stress level, and enhance your mental clarity.

Good Sleep: Getting a good night's sleep is crucial for boosting mental well-being, increasing vitality, and improving cognitive performance. The body goes through important processes, including hormone regulation, memory consolidation, and tissue repair. Aim for seven to nine hours of healthy sleep every night, and give appropriate sleep hygiene practices—like sticking to a regular sleep schedule, setting up a calming bedtime ritual, and making the most of your sleeping environment—first priority.

Handling Stress: Extended periods of stress can deplete one's energy reserves and hinder mental abilities, resulting in exhaustion, confusion, and reduced output. Stress levels may be lowered, relaxation can be encouraged, and mental clarity can be enhanced by engaging in stress-reduction practices such as progressive muscle relaxation, deep breathing, mindfulness, meditation, and yoga. Incorporating joyful and fulfilling activities into your life can also help mitigate the negative effects of stress and improve your general well-being.

The practice of mindful eating is being aware of the flavor, texture, and satiety signals of the meal while it is being consumed. You may better understand your body's signals of hunger and fullness, avoid overindulging, and enhance digestion by taking your time eating and enjoying every bite. Moreover, mindful eating may foster a positive relationship with food and increase one's enjoyment of it, which can boost one's energy and mental clarity.

Restricting Sugar and Caffeine: Although these substances might provide you with a short-term energy boost, using them too much will eventually cause energy collapses and poor mental clarity. Reducing the amount of sugary and caffeinated meals and beverages consumed can assist in maintaining energy levels and avoiding mood and cognitive repair, Instead, go for healthy options like fiber- and protein-rich snacks, water with lemon, or herbal teas.

Mental Health: Energy levels and mental clarity are directly related to mental well-being. Mood and mental clarity can be improved by taking part in activities that encourage connection, creativity, and relaxation. This might be going outside, cultivating thankfulness, engaging in hobbies, or spending time with close friends and family. Maintaining ideal energy levels and cognitive performance, as well as preventing burnout, may be achieved by taking periodic pauses throughout the day to rest and recharge.

Attaining and maintaining increased energy and mental clarity necessitates a comprehensive strategy that takes into account a variety of lifestyle factors, including nutrition, exercise, sleep, stress reduction, and mental health. People can optimize their energy and cognitive function, which leads to greater vitality and overall well-being, by prioritizing nutrient-dense foods, staying hydrated, exercising regularly, getting quality sleep, managing stress, practicing mindful eating, limiting caffeine and sugar intake, and fostering mental well-being. You may have steady energy and mental clarity throughout the day with self-care and consistency, which will help you succeed in all aspects of your life.

Taking care of chronic illnesses and diseases is a complicated and continuous process that calls for a multimodal strategy that includes continuing support, lifestyle changes, and medical care. Chronic illnesses, which include obesity, diabetes, heart disease, hypertension, autoimmune disorders, and other long-term problems, frequently need to be managed continuously in order to maximize quality of life and health. In this section, we'll examine several approaches and treatments for successfully controlling long-term illnesses and ailments:

Medical Care and Medication Administration: These two aspects of illness care are crucial for a number of chronic conditions. Prescription drugs to manage side effects, regulate symptoms, and halt the course of the illness may fall under this category. It's critical that people with chronic illnesses collaborate closely with their medical professionals to create individualized treatment programs that are suited to their unique requirements and objectives.

Frequent Monitoring and Health Assessments: Effective management of chronic illnesses and ailments depends on regular monitoring and health assessments. To determine the state of the condition, monitor its course, and assess the efficacy of therapy, routine check-ups, screenings, laboratory testing, and diagnostic procedures may be necessary. People may control their conditions and avoid problems by being proactive in managing their health by remaining knowledgeable about their condition.

Changes in Behavior and Lifestyle: Changing one's behavior and lifestyle is essential to treating chronic illnesses and disorders. This might entail forming healthy routines like consistent exercise, a balanced diet, stress reduction, getting enough sleep, abstaining from tobacco use, and limiting alcohol intake. Adopting sustainable lifestyle modifications can help alleviate symptoms, slow the course of the illness, and improve general health.

Nutrition Counseling and Dietary Management: These two key components are essential to the treatment of chronic illnesses, including obesity, diabetes, and heart disease. Making better food choices, navigating dietary restrictions, and creating customized meal plans are all made easier when people work with a licensed dietitian or nutritionist. Disease management and improved health outcomes can be achieved by placing an emphasis on nutrient-dense meals, portion control, and a balanced intake of macronutrients.

Programs for Physical Activity and Exercise: Managing chronic illnesses and conditions requires regular physical activity and exercise. Exercise supports weight control, strengthens bones and muscles, increases mobility, and improves cardiovascular health. It is recommended that individuals with chronic conditions collaborate with their healthcare practitioners to customize safe and suitable exercise regimens that are specific to their needs and current state of health.

Stress Reduction and Support for Mental Health: Long-term medical conditions can have a negative impact on one's mental and emotional health, increasing the risk of stress, anxiety, depression, and other mental health problems. An essential component of managing illness is stress management and placing a high priority on mental health. In order to foster emotional resilience and coping mechanisms, this may entail mindfulness exercises, psychotherapy, support groups, and other stress-reduction tactics.

Medication Adherence and Self-Management: For chronic illnesses and conditions to be properly managed, medication adherence and self-management are essential. This is adhering to treatment plans as provided, taking prescription drugs as instructed, keeping an eye on symptoms, and informing medical professionals of any changes or concerns. Participating in self-management activities encourages improved disease control and outcomes and gives people the power to actively manage their health.

Social Support and Community Resources: For those with chronic illnesses, social support and community resources may offer priceless help and encouragement. Family, friends, caregivers, support groups, organizations that advocate for patients, and community-based initiatives that provide information, resources, and peer support are a few examples of this. Developing a solid support system can help people manage the difficulties of having a chronic illness and enhance their general quality of life.

Ongoing Disease Management and Continued Education: Long-term successful management of chronic illnesses and diseases depends on ongoing disease management and continued education. This might entail routinely reviewing and modifying treatment plans as necessary, as well as keeping up to date on the most recent research, available treatments, and self-care techniques. Even when they have a chronic illness, people may still maximize their health and well-being by being proactive and involved in their healthcare.

Managing chronic illnesses and diseases calls for an all-encompassing, team-based strategy that takes continuing support, lifestyle changes, and medical treatment into account. Chronic disease and conditions can be effectively managed, quality of life improved, and complications reduced by individuals putting into practice strategies like medical treatment, regular monitoring, lifestyle modifications, dietary management, physical activity, stress reduction, medication adherence, social support, and ongoing education. Achieving good chronic illness management requires close collaboration with diet healthcare practitioners, taking part in self-management activities, and utilizing available resources and support networks.

a healthy

Improvements in digestive system and gut health

As it affects digestion, immunological response, food absorption, and even mental health, gut health is critical to overall health. Overall health is enhanced and proper digestive function is supported when the gut flora is in equilibrium. However, bad nutrition, stress, drugs, and lifestyle choices may all interfere with gut function, causing digestive problems and jeopardizing general health. Here, we'll discuss the significance of gut health as well as methods for enhancing digestive efficiency and fostering gut health:

Understanding Gut Health: The complex population of bacteria that live in the gastrointestinal system is referred to as the gut microbiota, also known as the gut microbiome. These microorganisms, which include viruses, fungi, bacteria, and other microbes, are essential for immune system development, metabolism, and digestion. A balanced gut microbiota promotes a healthy intestinal lining, controls inflammation, and aids in nutritional digestion and absorption.

Common Digestive Problems: Constipation, diarrhea, bloating, gas, GERD, IBS, and constipation are just a few of the common digestive problems that can seriously lower one's quality of life. Inflammation, dietary intolerances, abnormalities in the gut flora, and other factors frequently cause these problems. Enhancing gut health can help reduce symptoms related to digestion and improve general health.

Dietary interventions: Foods may either support or destroy a healthy gut microbiota. Dietary choices have a big impact on gut health. Prebiotics and probiotics from a diet high in fiber, fruits, vegetables, whole grains, and fermented foods enhance digestive health by feeding good gut flora. On the other hand, a diet heavy in sugar, refined carbs, processed foods, and bad fats can worsen gut health by encouraging inflammation and dysbiosis.

Foods High in Fiber: Fiber is necessary to maintain a healthy gut flora and to promote digestive health. Foods high in soluble fiber, such as legumes, fruits, and vegetables, function as prebiotics by nourishing good gut flora and encouraging regular bowel movements. Foods high in insoluble fiber, such as whole grains, nuts, seeds, and vegetables, help to promote a healthy digestive system and provide stool with more volume.

Fermented Foods: Packed with good probiotic bacteria, fermented foods can help mend the stomach lining. Yogurt, kefir, sauerkraut, kimchi, tempeh, and miso are examples of fermented foods that you may include in your diet to improve digestion, boost immunity, and introduce good bacteria into your gut.

Probiotic Supplements: If a person has digestive problems or an imbalance in their gut bacteria, probiotic supplements may also help to improve gut health. Live bacteria, known as probiotics, can improve gut microbiota balance and offer health advantages when taken in sufficient quantities. Seek out premium probiotic bacteria, cells that include a range of helpful bacterial strains and species.

Hydration: Sustaining gut health and preserving a healthy digestive system depends on getting enough water. Constipation may be avoided, and regular bowel movements and soft stool can be encouraged by consuming an ample amount of water. Try to obtain at least eight glasses of water each day, and to help with hydration and digestive health, think about eating foods high in water content, such as fruits and vegetables.

Stress management: Prolonged stress can have a deleterious effect on gut health by changing gut motility, raising inflammatory levels, and upsetting the microbiota's delicate equilibrium. Regular physical activity is beneficial for promoting gut health and supporting healthy digestion. Stress management techniques, such as mindfulness, meditation, deep breathing, yoga, and progressive muscle relaxation, can help reduce stress levels and support digestive health. Exercise promotes general well-being, lowers inflammation, and increases intestinal motility. Every day of the week, try to get in at least 30 minutes of moderate-intensity exercise to help your digestive system and general health.

Steer clear of trigger foods: Certain meals and drinks can aggravate stomach problems and interfere with gut function. Meals that are heavy in fat or sugar, artificial sweeteners, caffeine, alcohol, and spicy meals are common trigger foods. Keep an eye on how your body reacts to various meals, and steer clear of those that make you feel uncomfortable or cause stomach complaints.

Seeking Professional Advice: It's critical to seek professional advice from a healthcare physician or qualified dietitian if you're dealing with severe or persistent digestive problems. In order to promote gut health and enhance digestive function, they can offer individualized treatment suggestions, suggest suitable dietary and lifestyle changes, and assist in identifying the underlying reasons for digestive issues.

Health affects digestion, immunological response, nutritional absorption, and many other aspects of general health. Through the application of tactics including eating a well-balanced diet high in fiber and fermented foods, drinking plenty of water, controlling stress, exercising frequently, and avoiding trigger foods, people may maintain gut health and encourage a balanced microbiota. Additionally, getting expert advice from medical professionals or qualified dietitians might result in tailored suggestions for treating certain digestive problems and enhancing gut health. People can boost general well-being, reduce symptoms, and improve digestive function with proactive treatment and lifestyle measures.

Hormonal equilibrium and metabolic well-being

The body's many physiological functions are regulated by both hormonal balance and metabolic health, which are intimately related. Hormones are chemical messengers that regulate metabolism, development, reproduction, and stress responses, among other processes. A disturbed hormonal balance can result in weight gain, insulin resistance, metabolic malfunction, and other health problems. We'll discuss the significance of hormonal balance and metabolic health here, along with methods for enhancing each:

Understanding Hormonal Balance: The proper interaction and control of different hormones inside the body is referred to as hormonal balance. Endocrine glands, which include the pituitary, thyroid, adrenal, pancreatic, ovarian, and testicular, are responsible for producing hormones. Target tissues and organs are affected by these hormones' actions, which also affect blood sugar balance, energy generation, metabolism, and other physiological processes.

Important Hormones: A number of important hormones are essential for controlling metabolic health. These consist of leptin, ghrelin, adrenaline, estrogen, progesterone, testosterone, glucagon, cortisol, and thyroid hormones (T3 and T4). Every hormone in the body has a distinct purpose, and when any of these hormones are out of balance, it can cause metabolic problems and other health problems.

Metabolic Health: When there is optimal metabolic function, blood sugar levels are steady, energy generation is efficient, weight management is healthy, and lipid profiles are normal. Hormone balance, genetics, physical activity, stress, food, and sleep quality are some of the variables that affect metabolic health. The chance of developing chronic illnesses including type 2 diabetes, obesity, cardiovascular disease, and metabolic syndrome might rise when metabolic health is disturbed.

Hormonal imbalance's Effect on Metabolic Health: Imbalances in hormones have a major effect on metabolic health and can even lead to metabolic dysfunction. As an illustration, insulin resistance, a disorder in which cells lose their sensitivity to insulin, can result in high blood sugar, weight gain, and a higher chance of type 2 diabetes. Thyroid hormone abnormalities can also impair metabolism and cause symptoms including weariness, fluctuations in body weight, and trouble controlling body temperature.

Nutrition and diet: Nutrition and diet are essential for maintaining hormonal balance and metabolic health. In addition to providing vital nutrients and supporting hormone synthesis and control, eating a balanced diet full of whole foods, such as fruits, vegetables, lean proteins, healthy fats, and complex carbs, is important. Preventing insulin spikes, inflammation, and hormone imbalances can be achieved by avoiding processed meals, refined carbohydrates, and unhealthy fats.

Blood Sugar Regulation: Hormonal balance and metabolic health depend on blood sugar regulation. Eating low-glycemic meals, such as legumes, whole grains, and non-starchy vegetables, can help avoid insulin resistance and normalize blood sugar levels. Eating healthy, balanced meals and snacks on a regular basis can also help control blood sugar levels and avoid energy slumps.

Physical Activity and Exercise: Maintaining hormone balance and metabolic health requires regular physical activity and exercise. Exercise improves cell absorption of glucose, raises insulin sensitivity, and speeds up the burning of fat. To maximize hormone balance and metabolic health, try to incorporate strength training, flexibility training, and cardiovascular activity.

Stress management: prolonged stress raises cortisol levels, fuels inflammation, and exacerbates insulin resistance, all of which can upset hormonal balance and metabolic health. Reducing stress and promoting hormone balance can be achieved by putting stress-reduction strategies such as progressive muscle relaxation, deep breathing, mindfulness, meditation, and yoga into practice.

Sleep Quality: Hormonal balance and metabolic health depend on getting enough sleep. Hormones that control hunger and metabolism, such as cortisol, leptin, and ghrelin, might be produced inefficiently or poorly. Aim for 7–9 hours of good sleep each night to maintain the best possible hormonal and metabolic balance.

Steer clear of environmental toxins: Endocrine-disrupting chemicals (EDCs), which are present in plastics, insecticides, and personal hygiene items, are examples of environmental pollutants that can disrupt hormone synthesis and control, resulting in metabolic dysfunction. Hormone balance and metabolic health can be supported by minimizing exposure to these chemicals through the use of natural cleaning and personal care products, avoiding plastic containers, and choosing organic foods.

Medical Management and Hormone Treatment: To enhance metabolic health and restore hormonal balance, medical management and hormone treatment may be required in specific circumstances. This might involve thyroid hormone replacement treatment, blood sugar-regulating drugs, or hormone replacement therapy for people deficient in testosterone, progesterone, or estrogen. Selecting the best course of action for a patient's requirements and health requires close collaboration with medical professionals.

For general health and the best possible functioning of the body, hormonal balance and metabolic health are critical. Individuals may maintain hormonal balance and enhance metabolic health by adopting good lifestyle behaviors, such as a balanced diet, frequent exercise, stress management, enough sleep, and avoiding environmental contaminants. Additionally, hormonal abnormalities may be addressed, and metabolic function can be optimized by obtaining medical advice and therapy as necessary. People can improve their metabolic health, attain hormonal balance, and live better overall with proactive management and lifestyle modifications.

Carnivore Waffles

Introduction: Carnivore waffles offer a delightful twist to your breakfast routine, providing a high-protein start to your day without any carbs. This dish is especially suitable for those following a strict carnivore diet, looking for variety in their meal plans.

Ingredients:

4 eggs

2 tablespoons of cream cheese (ensure it's full-fat)

1 tablespoon of butter (for greasing the waffle iron)

Preparation Time: 15 minutes

Instructions:

Preheat your waffle iron and grease it with butter.

Blend the eggs and cream cheese together until the mixture is smooth.

Pour the batter into the waffle iron and cook according to the iron's instructions, usually about 3-5 minutes, until the waffle is golden and slightly crispy.

Serve hot.

Health Benefits: Eggs are a fantastic source of high-quality protein and essential nutrients, which are pivotal for muscle maintenance and overall health. Cream cheese adds a bit of fat, which can help to keep you full and satisfied.

Importance in Diet: This recipe provides a fulfilling meal that supports a zero-carb lifestyle, helping to maintain energy levels without spiking blood sugar.

Cheesy Carnivore Omelets

Introduction: Starting your day with a Cheesy Carnivore Omelet can bring comfort and satisfaction. It's not only delicious but packed with nutrients essential for body function and health.

Ingredients:

3 eggs

1/2 cup shredded cheddar cheese

2 tablespoons of butter or animal fat

Salt to taste (optional)

Preparation Time: 10 minutes

Instructions:

Beat the eggs in a bowl and set aside.

Heat butter in a non-stick skillet over medium heat.

Pour the eggs into the skillet, letting them sit until they start to set around the edges.

Sprinkle the shredded cheese over the eggs.

Fold the omelet in half and continue to cook until the cheese is melted and the eggs are cooked to your preference.

Serve immediately.

Health Benefits: Eggs are rich in protein and essential vitamins, while cheese provides calcium for bone health and fats for energy.

Importance in Diet: This dish supports muscle function and bone health, and the high fat content helps to keep you feeling full, aiding in weight management and satiety throughout the day.

Pancake Patties

Introduction: Pancake Patties are a unique and savory take on traditional breakfast pancakes, adapted for those on a carnivore diet. They are simple, nutritious, and a comforting way to enjoy a familiar breakfast favorite without the carbs.

Ingredients:

1 pound ground beef

2 eggs

Salt and pepper to taste

Preparation Time: 20 minutes

Instructions:

Preheat a skillet over medium heat.

In a bowl, mix the ground beef, eggs, salt, and pepper until well combined.

Form the mixture into small, thin patties.

Cook the patties in the skillet for about 3-4 minutes on each side, or until fully cooked.

Serve hot.

Health Benefits: Ground beef is an excellent source of protein and iron, which are crucial for muscle growth and maintaining healthy blood cells. Eggs add additional protein and nutrients.

Importance in Diet: Pancake patties provide a hearty, protein-rich meal that supports muscle building and energy levels, aligning well with the carnivore diet's emphasis on high-protein, low-carb foods.

Breakfast Sandwich for Carnivores

Introduction: Start your day off right with a hearty Carnivore Breakfast Sandwich. This recipe makes your morning process easier and fits with the carnivore diet's high-protein, low-carb rules.

Ingredients:

2 big eggs

Two bacon or ham slices

One piece of cheddar cheese

Add salt and pepper to taste.

Five minutes to get ready.

Cooking Time: 10 minutes

15 minutes all together

Instructions:

Cook the Bacon/Ham: In a pan over medium heat, cook the bacon until crispy or the ham until lightly browned. Remove and set away on a paper towel.

Fry the Eggs: Fry the eggs in the same skillet to your desired doneness. Season with salt and pepper.

Assemble: Layer one egg on a plate, top with cheese, bacon or ham, and then the second egg. Use the eggs as buns for a zero-carb sandwich.

Health Benefits:

This sandwich is packed with high-quality protein and fats, important for muscle maintenance and overall health. It's perfect for those trying to stay in ketosis.

Dietary Importance: This fulfilling breakfast sets a strong base for energy levels and satiety throughout the day, supporting your strict dietary commitments.

Carnivore Fat Bomb Fluffy Egg & Cheese Muffins

Introduction: Ideal for a snack or a quick meal, these fluffy muffins are a lovely way to keep your energy up without any carbs.

Ingredients

6 large eggs

1/2 cup shredded cheddar cheese

1/4 cup finely chopped cooked bacon

Add salt and pepper to taste.

Five minutes to get ready.

Cooking Time: 15 minutes

Total Time: 20 minutes

Instructions:

Preheat the oven: Heat your oven to 350°F (175°C).

Combine Ingredients: In a bowl, whisk the eggs with salt and pepper. Stir in the cheese and bacon.

Bake: Pour the batter into greased muffin tins and bake for 15 minutes, or until the muffins are firm and golden.

Health Benefits: These muffins are a great source of fats and proteins, aiding in muscle repair and giving lasting energy.

Dietary Importance: They're a convenient, portable choice that fits well into a meal-prep routine, supporting your dietary goals on busy days.

Two-Ingredient Carnivore Pancakes

Introduction: Sometimes simplicity is key, especially when following a strict diet. These two-ingredient pancakes are incredibly easy to make and surprisingly filling.

Ingredients:

4 large eggs

4 ounces cream cheese, softened

Five minutes to get ready.

Cooking Time: 5 minutes per batch

Total Time: 10 minutes

Instructions:

Blend Ingredients: Blend the eggs and cream cheese until smooth.

Cook: Pour small amounts of the batter onto a hot, greased pan. Cook for 2-3 minutes on each side until golden brown.

Health Benefits: These pancakes are low in carbs and high in fat, making them ideal for maintaining ketosis and energy levels.

Dietary Importance: Perfect for breakfast or as a snack, they help you adhere to your carnivore dietary commitments while having a treat.

Introduction: Start your day with Carnivore Diet Breakfast Tacos, a creative twist on traditional breakfast that keeps carbs to a minimum while maximizing taste and protein intake.

Ingredients:

4 large eggs

4 slices of ham (used as the taco shells)

1 cup cooked ground beef or sausage

Salt and pepper to taste

Optional: Cheese for topping

Preparation Time: 10 minutes

Cooking Time: 10 minutes

Total Time: 20 minutes

Instructions:

Cook the Meat: Brown your ground beef or sausage in a pan until fully cooked. Season with salt and pepper.

Prepare the Eggs: In another pan, scramble the eggs until just set.

Heat the Ham: Briefly warm the ham slices in the pan to make them pliable.

Assemble the Tacos: Use the ham pieces as taco shells. Spoon some beaten eggs and ground meat into each ham slice, folding gently.

Serve: Top with cheese if desired and serve quickly.

Health Benefits: Packed with high-quality protein, these breakfast tacos support muscle repair and growth and provide steady energy levels throughout the morning.

Dietary Importance: This breakfast option is ideal for those on a strict carnivore diet, giving a fulfilling and satisfying start to the day without any carbs.

Introduction: Creamy Shrimp and Eggs is a luxurious yet simple dish, great for a high-protein start to the day or a delightful brunch.

Instructions

8 big shrimp, peeled and deveined

4 eggs

1/4 cup heavy cream

2 tablespoons unsalted butter

Salt and pepper to taste

Five minutes to get ready.

Cooking Time: 10 minutes

15 minutes all together

Instructions:

Cook the Shrimp: Melt butter in a pan over medium heat. Add the shrimp and cook until pink and opaque, about 2-3 minutes per side.

Scramble the Eggs: In a bowl, mix together eggs, heavy cream, salt, and pepper. Pour over the cooked shrimp in the pan, stirring gently until the eggs are softly set.

Serve: Serve hot, garnished with a sprinkle of fresh herbs if wanted.

Health Benefits: This dish is rich in proteins and fats, which are necessary for brain function and maintaining energy levels. Shrimp offers a high amount of selenium and vitamin B12.

Dietary Importance: The combination of shrimp and eggs provides a nutritious meal that fits well within the parameters of the carnivore diet, boosting general health and well-being.

Carnivore Casserole

Introduction: Carnivore Casserole is a hearty, meaty dish that's great for dinner or as a satiating meal at any time of the day, packed with various meats to keep you full and satisfied.

Things used:

1 pound ground beef

1/2 pound bacon, chopped

1/2 pound sausage, crumbled 4 eggs

1/2 cup heavy cream

Salt and pepper to taste

Optional: Shredded cheese for topping

Preparation Time: 15 minutes

Cooking Time: 30 minutes

Total Time: 45 minutes

Instructions:

Preheat the oven: Preheat your oven to 350°F (175°C).

Cook the Meats: In a big skillet, cook the bacon and sausage until browned. Add ground beef and cook until no pink remains.

Prepare the Egg Mixture: In a bowl, mix together the eggs, heavy cream, salt, and pepper.

Assemble the casserole: In a serving dish, layer the cooked meats. Pour the egg mixture over the meat.

Bake: Bake in the preheated oven for 25-30 minutes, or until the eggs are set and the top is golden brown. Add cheese and bake for an additional 5 minutes if using.

Serve: Let it cool slightly before serving.

Health Benefits: This casserole is an excellent source of protein and fat, important for energy and satiety. It helps muscle maintenance and growth.

Dietary Importance: Ideal for those strictly following the carnivore diet, this dish makes meal prep easy.

Introduction: Herby's Bone Broth is a nourishing and flavorful base for any carnivore's diet. It combines the profound benefits of bone broth with a slight hint of herbs, making it a perfect standalone warm drink or a base for other recipes.

Ingredients:

2 pounds of mixed bones (beef, chicken, or pork)

1 gallon of water

2 tablespoons apple cider vinegar

Herbs (optional, such as thyme or rosemary for taste)

Salt to taste

Preparation Time: 10 minutes

Cooking Time: 12-24 hours

Total Time: Up to 24 hours and 10 minutes

Instructions:

Prepare the Bones: Place the bones in a big pot or slow cooker. Add the apple cider vinegar and water. The vinegar helps remove nutrients from the bones.

Slow Cook: Bring to a simmer, lower the heat, and cover. Allow to cook for 12-24 hours. The longer you cook, the more flavorful and healthy the broth.

Add Herbs: In the last hour of cooking, add any optional herbs for added flavor.

Strain and Season: Strain the soup through a fine-mesh sieve and discard the solids. Season with salt to taste.

Store or Serve: Serve warm or store in the refrigerator for up to 5 days.

Health Benefits:

Rich in minerals and collagen, bone broth benefits joint health, digestive health, and skin elasticity. It's a comforting, immune-boosting food great for any diet, especially during colder months.

Dietary Importance: Herby's Bone Broth is a versatile component of the carnivore diet, providing important nutrients that are hard to obtain from muscle meats alone.

Keto Carnivore Waffles

Introduction: Keto Carnivore Waffles offer a delightful twist on a breakfast favorite, using ingredients compliant with a ketogenic carnivore diet. They are great for those looking for low-carb, high-protein alternatives to traditional waffles.

Ingredients:

4 eggs

1 cup of ground pork rinds (as a replacement for flour)

1/2 cup shredded cheese

1/4 cup heavy cream

Butter or oil for greasing the waffle iron

Five minutes to get ready.

Cooking Time: 5 minutes

Total Time: 10 minutes

Instructions:

Blend Ingredients: In a blender, add eggs, ground pork rinds, shredded cheese, and heavy cream until smooth.

Preheat Waffle Iron: Preheat your waffle iron and grease it with butter or oil.

Cook: Pour the batter into the waffle iron and cook according to the manufacturer's guidelines, usually about 3-5 minutes, until golden and crispy.

Serve: Serve hot with butter or your choice of carnivore-friendly toppings.

Health Benefits: These waffles are rich in protein and fats, making them satiating and ideal for energy digestion. The absence of grains and sugars helps control blood sugar levels.

Dietary Importance: A creative and enjoyable way to vary meals within the carnivore diet, these waffles can help you feel satisfied and catered to, even on a restrictive diet.

3 Ingredient Carnivore Custard

Introduction: 3 Ingredient Carnivore Custard is a simple, creamy dessert that fits nicely into a carnivore diet plan. It's easy to make and can fill your dessert cravings without breaking dietary rules.

Ingredient:

6 egg yolks

1 cup thick cream

Sweetener (optional, consider a carnivore-friendly choice if needed)

Five minutes to get ready.

Cooking Time: 10 minutes

15 minutes all together

Instructions:

Mix Ingredients: In a mixing bowl, whisk together the egg whites, heavy cream, and sweetener if using.

Cook on Low Heat: Pour the mixture into a pot. Cook over low heat, stirring constantly, until the liquid thickens enough to coat the back of a spoon.

Chill: Remove from heat and pour the custard into a bowl. Cover and chill in the refrigerator until set, about 2 hours.

Serve: Serve chilled, plain, or with a sprinkle of cinnamon or nutmeg if wanted.

Health Benefits: This custard is rich in fats.

Carnivore Quiche

Introduction: Carnivore Quiche offers a delightful variation by focusing completely on animal products. It's a perfect dish for any meal, giving both nourishment and satisfaction without any carbs.

Ingredients:

6 eggs

1 cup thick cream

1 cup cooked bacon, chopped

1 cup shredded cheese (such as cheddar or gouda)

Salt and pepper to taste. Preparation Time: 10 minutes

Cooking Time: 35 minutes

Total Time: 45 minutes

Instructions:

Preheat the oven: Preheat your oven to 350°F (175°C).

Mix Ingredients: In a large bowl, mix together the eggs and heavy cream. Stir in the cooked bacon, cheese, and season with salt and pepper.

Prepare the Dish: Pour the mixture into a greased pie dish.

Bake: Place in the oven and bake for 35 minutes, or until the quiche is set and the top is golden brown.

Serve: Allow to cool slightly before slicing. Serve warm.

Health Benefits: This quiche is rich in proteins and fats, which are necessary for building and maintaining muscle mass, and supporting cellular functions.

Dietary Importance: Adapting to a strict carnivore diet can be difficult, but this quiche makes it enjoyable, providing a comforting and filling meal that perfectly aligns with dietary restrictions.

Introduction: Salmon steak is not only a culinary delight but also a powerhouse of nutrition, perfect for a carnivore diet looking to add healthy fats and high-quality proteins.

Ingredient:

2 salmon steaks (about 6 ounces each)

2 tablespoons olive oil or melted butter

Salt and pepper to taste

Lemon wedges (optional, for serving)

Five minutes to get ready.

Cooking Time: 10 minutes

15 minutes all together

Instructions:

Prepare the salmon: Pat the salmon steaks dry with paper towels. Season both sides with salt and pepper.

Heat the Oil/Butter: In a pan over medium-high heat, heat the olive oil or butter.

Cook the Salmon: Place the salmon steaks in the pan. Cook for about 5 minutes on each side, or until the salmon is fully cooked and flakes easily with a fork.

Serve: Serve hot, with lemon wedges if wanted for added flavor.

Health Benefits: Salmon is rich in omega-3 fatty acids, which are important for cardiovascular health, brain function, and reducing inflammation.

Dietary Importance: Incorporating salmon into your diet provides important nutrients that support a healthy metabolism and can help maintain weight management goals on a carnivore diet.

Meatloaf

Introduction: This Carnivore Meatloaf strips back the traditional recipe to its meaty core, focusing on high-protein ingredients for a satisfying and hearty meal.

Ingredients:

2 pounds ground beef

2 eggs

1 cup grated Parmesan cheese

2 tablespoons Worcestershire sauce (ensure it's sugar-free for true carnivore compliance)

Salt and pepper to taste Preparation Time: 15 minutes

Cooking Time: 1 hour

Total Time: 1 hour, 15 minutes

Instructions:

Preheat the oven: Preheat your oven to 350°F (175°C).

Combine Ingredients: In a big bowl, mix together the ground beef, eggs, Parmesan, Worcestershire sauce, salt, and pepper.

Shape the meatloaf: Transfer the mixture to a bread pan or shape it into a loaf on a baking sheet.

Bake: Place in the oven and bake for about 1 hour, or until the meatloaf is cooked through and the top is browned.

Serve: Let it rest for a few minutes before slicing. Serve warm.

Health Benefits: Meatloaf is a great source of high-quality protein, which is necessary for muscle repair and growth. The added eggs and cheese boost the meal's nutrient value.

Dietary Importance:: This meal is a cornerstone for those following a carnivore diet, providing a fulfilling and protein-rich dish that can be enjoyed at any time, ensuring adherence to dietary goals.

Sausages and Scrambled Eggs

Introduction: Sausages and scrambled eggs are a standard breakfast combo that packs a protein punch to start your day off right. This meal is quick to prepare and offers the energy and satiety needed to handle your morning activities.

Ingredients:

4 large eggs

4 sausages (choose a type compatible with your dietary needs)

2 tablespoons of milk or cream (optional, for fluffier eggs)

Salt and pepper to taste

Butter or oil for cooking

Five minutes to get ready.

Cooking Time: 10 minutes

15 minutes all together

Instructions:

Cook the Sausages: In a skillet over medium heat, cook the sausages until browned and cooked through, turning regularly. This usually takes about 8-10 minutes.

Prepare Scrambled Eggs: While sausages are cooking, whisk the eggs with milk (if using), salt, and pepper. In another pan, heat a knob of butter or a splash of oil, pour in the eggs, and cook, stirring frequently, until they are softly set.

Serve: Slice the sausages if wanted and serve alongside the scrambled eggs.

Health Benefits: This meal is rich in protein, which is important for muscle repair and growth. The fats in the eggs and sausages provide prolonged energy without spiking blood sugar levels.

Dietary Importance: For those on a low-carb or ketogenic diet, this breakfast is ideal for staying within macro limits while giving lasting fullness and energy.

Introduction: An Egg and Protein Shake is a supercharged start to your day, mixing high-quality protein in a quick, drinkable form. It's especially good for those times when you need a quick boost before heading out the door.

Ingredients:

1 raw egg (ensure it's good quality and very fresh)

1 scoop of your favorite protein powder

1 cup of almond milk or water

Ice cubes (optional)

Preparation Time: 2 minutes

Total Time: 2 minutes

Instructions:

Combine Ingredients: In a blender, add the raw egg, protein powder, almond milk or water, and ice cubes.

Blend: Blend on high until smooth and bubbly.

Serve: Pour into a glass and drink quickly for the best flavor and nutrient intake.

Health Benefits: Packed with protein, this shake helps muscle synthesis and recovery. It's also quick to digest, making it great for post-workout replenishment.

Dietary Importance: This shake is a fantastic way to get a concentrated dose of protein without any fuss, aligning well with fitness goals and busy lives.

Bacon and Eggs

Introduction: Bacon and Eggs is a classic breakfast that's beloved for its simplicity and satisfying nature. This dish is a staple in low-carb diets due to its high protein and fat content.

Ingredient:

4 slices of bacon

4 eggs

Salt and pepper to taste

Butter or oil for cooking

Five minutes to get ready.

Cooking Time: 10 minutes

15 minutes all together

Instructions:

Cook the Bacon: In a pan over medium heat, cook the bacon until crispy, about 5-7 minutes. Remove and set aside on paper towels to dry.

Fry the Eggs: In the same skillet, use the bacon grease to fry the eggs to your chosen doneness. Season with salt and pepper.

Serve: Serve the eggs with the crispy bacon.

Health Benefits: Bacon and eggs offer a good mix of protein and fats, which can help regulate hunger hormones and blood sugar levels throughout the morning.

Dietary Importance: This meal fits perfectly within a ketogenic or carnivore diet, giving important nutrients to start the day without any carbohydrates.

Sausages and Scrambled Eggs

Introduction: Sausages and scrambled eggs is a standard breakfast combo that packs a protein punch to start your day off right. This meal is quick to prepare and offers the energy and satiety needed to handle your morning activities.

Ingredients:

4 large eggs

4 sausages (choose a type compatible with your dietary needs)

2 tablespoons of milk or cream (optional, for fluffier eggs)

Salt and pepper to taste

Butter or oil for cooking

Five minutes to get ready.

Cooking Time: 10 minutes

15 minutes all together

Instructions:

Cook the Sausages: In a skillet over medium heat, cook the sausages until browned and cooked through, turning regularly. This usually takes about 8-10 minutes.

Prepare Scrambled Eggs: While sausages are cooking, whisk the eggs with milk (if using), salt, and pepper. In another pan, heat a knob of butter or a splash of oil, pour in the eggs, and cook, stirring frequently, until they are softly set.

Serve: Slice the sausages if wanted and serve alongside the scrambled eggs.

Health Benefits: This meal is rich in protein, which is important for muscle repair and growth. The fats in the eggs and sausages provide prolonged energy without spiking blood sugar levels.

Dietary Importance: For those on a low-carb or ketogenic diet, this breakfast is ideal for staying within macro limits while giving lasting fullness and energy.

Egg and Protein Shake

Introduction: An Egg and Protein Shake is a supercharged start to your day, mixing high-quality protein in a quick, drinkable form. It's especially good for those times when you need a quick boost before heading out the door.

Ingredients:

1 raw egg (ensure it's good quality and very fresh)

1 scoop of your favorite protein powder

1 cup of almond milk or water

Ice cubes (optional)

Preparation Time: 2 minutes

Total Time: 2 minutes

Instructions:

Combine Ingredients: In a blender, add the raw egg, protein powder, almond milk or water, and ice cubes.

Blend: Blend on high until smooth and bubbly.

Serve: Pour into a glass and drink quickly for the best flavor and nutrient intake.

Health Benefits: Packed with protein, this shake helps muscle synthesis and recovery. It's also quick to digest, making it great for post-workout replenishment.

Dietary Importance: This shake is a fantastic way to get a concentrated dose of protein without any fuss, aligning well with fitness goals and busy lives.

Scrambled Lamb Brain and Eggs

Introduction: Scrambled Lamb Brain and Eggs is a nutrient-dense dish that taps into traditional delicacies, providing an excellent source of omega-3 fatty acids and cholesterol, which are important for brain health.

Ingredients:

1 lamb brain, cleaned and finely chopped

4 eggs

2 tablespoons butter

Salt and pepper to taste. Preparation Time: 10 minutes

Cooking Time: 10 minutes

Total Time: 20 minutes

Instructions:

Prepare the Brain: Soak the lamb brain in cold water for an hour to remove any blood. Drain and carefully remove the covering. Chop finely.

Cook the Brain: In a pan, melt 1 tablespoon of butter over medium heat. Add the chopped brain and sauté for about 3-4 minutes until lightly cooked.

Add Eggs: Beat the eggs with salt and pepper. Pour over the lamb brain in the pan. Stir gently to mix as the eggs cook and scramble.

Serve: Once the eggs are fully cooked, remove from heat. Serve hot, garnished with herbs if wanted.

Nutritional Benefits: Lamb brain is rich in omega-3 fatty acids, which are necessary for brain function and overall cellular health. Eggs provide high-quality protein and vitamins.

Dietary Importance: This dish is particularly beneficial for those on a carnivore diet looking to enhance their nutrient intake, especially important brain nutrients not usually found in muscle meats.

Introduction: A properly seared steak is not just a meal; it's an experience. Rich in protein, iron, and B vitamins, it's a classic part of any carnivore's diet.

Ingredients:

2 ribeye or sirloin steaks (about 1-inch thick)

Salt and ground black pepper

2 tablespoons olive oil or butter

Five minutes to get ready.

Cooking Time: 10 minutes

15 minutes all together

Instructions:

Preheat pan: Heat a cast-iron pan over high heat. Add the olive oil or butter.

Prepare the Steak: Season the steaks heavily with salt and pepper.

Sear the Steak: Place the steaks in the hot pan. Cook for about 4-5 minutes on each side for medium-rare, or adjust according to your taste.

Rest the Steak: Remove the steaks from the pan and let them rest for about 5 minutes before serving. This helps keep the juices flowing.

Nutritional Benefits: Steak is an excellent source of high-quality protein, iron, and important B vitamins necessary for energy and overall health.

Dietary Importance: Including steak in your diet can help maintain muscle mass and strength, which are important for a healthy metabolism on a carnivore diet.

Carnivore Egg-in-a-Hole

Introduction: Carnivore Egg-in-a-Hole reinvents a standard breakfast with a purely carnivorous twist, using meat as the "bread" base.

Ingredients:

4 big slices of ham or thick-cut bacon

4 eggs

Salt and pepper to taste

Butter or oil for cooking

Five minutes to get ready.

Cooking Time: 10 minutes

15 minutes all together

Instructions:

Prepare the meat: If using bacon, partly cook it until it's flexible but not crispy. If using ham, use it as is.

Cook the Egg-in-a-Hole: In a pan, heat butter or oil. Place the meat slices and carefully crack an egg into the center of each piece. Season with salt and pepper.

Finish Cooking: Cook over medium heat until the egg whites are set and the yolks are cooked to your liking.

Nutritional Benefits: This dish combines high-quality protein and fats from both eggs and meat, giving a sustained energy source and essential nutrients.

Dietary Importance: A playful twist on traditional breakfasts, this dish fits with the carnivore diet's principles while keeping meals interesting and flavorful.

Carnivore Breakfast Muffins

Introduction: Carnivore Breakfast Muffins make a great grab-and-go breakfast or snack, packed with protein and fats to fuel your day without any carbs.

Ingredients:

6 eggs

1/2 pound ground sausage or bacon, cooked and crumbled

1 cup shredded cheddar cheese

Salt and pepper to taste.

Preparation Time: 10 minutes

Cooking Time: 15 minutes

Total Time: 25 minutes

Instructions:

Preheat Oven: Heat your oven to 350°F (175°C) and grease a muffin pan.

Mix Ingredients: In a bowl, whisk the eggs and mix in the cooked sausage or bacon, cheese, and a pinch of salt and pepper.

Fill Muffin Tin: Spoon the batter into the muffin cups, filling each about three-quarters full.

Bake: Place in the oven and bake for 15 minutes, or until the eggs are set and the tops are slightly yellow.

Serve: Remove from the oven, let cool slightly, and serve warm.

Nutritional Benefits: These muffins are high in protein and fat, which can help maintain muscle mass and satiety, crucial for those on a carnivore diet.

Dietary Importance: Easy to make and portable, these muffins fit perfectly into a busy lifestyle, ensuring adherence to dietary restrictions without sacrificing ease or taste.

Three Cheese Omelette

Introduction: This Three Cheese Omelette is a cheesy treat that brings together the rich flavors of different cheeses in a fluffy egg base, making a satisfying meal any time of the day.

Ingredients:

3 large eggs

1/4 cup grated cheddar cheese

1/4 cup grated mozzarella cheese

1/4 cup grated Parmesan cheese

2 tablespoons butter

Salt and pepper to taste Preparation Time: 5 minutes

Cooking Time: 5 minutes

Total Time: 10 minutes

Instructions:

Beat the Eggs: In a bowl, beat the eggs with salt and pepper.

Heat the butter: In a non-stick pan, melt the butter over medium heat.

Cook the Omelette: Pour the eggs into the pan. As the edges start to set, slowly pull them towards the center, allowing the uncooked eggs to flow to the edges.

Add Cheese: Sprinkle the cheddar, mozzarella, and Parmesan equally over the eggs. Let cook until the eggs are set and the cheese is melted.

Fold and Serve: Carefully fold the omelette in half and slide onto a plate to serve.

Nutritional Benefits: Loaded with high-quality protein and calcium, this omelette benefits bone health and muscle function.

Dietary Importance: A cheese omelette offers a fulfilling way to start the day, giving sustained energy and important nutrients within the constraints of a carnivore diet.

Carnivore Casserole with Ground Beef

Introduction: Carnivore Casserole with Ground Beef is a hearty, meaty dish that's both nourishing and comforting, great for dinner or as a meal prep solution.

Ingredients:

2 pounds ground beef

1 cup beef broth; 1 cup shredded cheese (optional, for topping)

1/2 cup heavy cream

2 eggs

Salt and pepper to taste

Preparation Time: 15 minutes

Cooking Time: 30 minutes

Total Time: 45 minutes

Instructions:

Preheat the oven: Preheat your oven to 375°F (190°C).

Brown the Beef: In a pan, cook the ground beef until browned. Season with salt and pepper. Drain any extra fat.

Mix Ingredients: In a bowl, whisk together the eggs, heavy cream, and beef stock. Add the cooked beef and mix well.

Assemble the Casserole: Transfer the beef mixture to a baking dish. Top with shredded cheese if using.

Bake: Bake in the preheated oven for about 30 minutes, or until the batter is bubbly and the top is golden brown.

Serve: Let the dish cool for a few minutes before serving.

Nutritional Benefits: This casserole is rich in protein, essential fats, and good protein

Introduction: Steak and eggs are a classic combination that provides a powerhouse of proteins and nutrients, perfect for starting the day with strength or recovering after a workout.

Ingredients:

2 ribeye or sirloin steaks (about 6 ounces each)

4 large eggs

Salt and pepper to taste

2 tablespoons butter or oil

Five minutes to get ready.

Cooking Time: 15 minutes

Total Time: 20 minutes

Instructions:

Prepare the Steak: Season the steaks with salt and pepper. Heat a pan over medium-high heat and add one tablespoon of butter or oil. Sear the steaks for about 4-5 minutes on each side for medium-rare, or adjust to your taste. Remove it from the pan and let it rest.

Cook the eggs: In the same pan, add another tablespoon of butter or oil. Crack the eggs into the pan and fry to your liking.

Serve: Slice the steak and serve alongside the fried eggs.

Nutritional Benefits: This meal is rich in high-quality protein, which is important for muscle repair and growth. The fats from the steak and eggs are great for hormone release and provide lasting energy.

Dietary Importance: Steak and eggs represent the principles of the carnivore diet, focusing on animal-based foods to support a low-carb, high-protein regimen that aids in keeping muscle mass and reducing cravings.

Carnivore Egg Pudding

Introduction: Carnivore Egg Pudding is a simple, creamy dessert that sticks to the carnivore diet while satisfying your sweet tooth in a healthy way.

Ingredients:

6 large eggs

1 cup thick cream

Sweetener to taste (optional, use a carnivore-friendly sweetener if preferred)

Five minutes to get ready.

Cooking Time: 10 minutes

15 minutes all together

Instructions:

Blend Ingredients: In a blender, add eggs, heavy cream, and sweetener if using. Blend until smooth.

Cook: Pour the mixture into a saucepan and cook over low heat, stirring constantly, until the mixture thickens to a pudding-like consistency.

Chill: Pour the pudding into bowls and chill in the refrigerator until set, about 2 hours.

Serve: Enjoy chilled, garnished with a sprinkle of cinnamon or nutmeg, if preferred.

Nutritional Benefits: Eggs and cream are excellent sources of protein and healthy fats, contributing to brain health and overall satiety.

Dietary Importance: This pudding allows those on the carnivore diet to enjoy a dessert that fits within their dietary restrictions, giving a satisfying and nutritious end to a meal.

Savory Brisket Queso

Introduction: Savory Brisket Queso combines rich, tender brisket with creamy, melted cheese, creating a deliciously indulgent dish that's great for dipping or as a hearty meal on its own.

Ingredients:

1 pound cooked beef, shredded

1 cup thick cream

2 cups shredded cheddar cheese

1/2 teaspoon smoked paprika (optional)

Salt to taste

Preparation Time: 10 minutes

Cooking Time: 10 minutes

Total Time: 20 minutes

Instructions:

Heat Ingredients: In a saucepan over medium heat, mix the heavy cream and shredded cheese. Stir until the cheese is melted and the mixture is smooth.

Add Brisket: Stir in the chopped brisket and smoked paprika if using. Continue to cook, stirring frequently, until the meat is heated through.

Season and Serve: Season with salt to taste. Serve warm with a side of more carnivore-friendly choices, such as pork rinds or homemade meat chips.

Nutritional Benefits: This food is high in protein and fats, making it very satiating. The brisket provides iron and B vitamins, which are necessary for energy metabolism.

Dietary Importance: Savory Brisket Queso is a flexible dish that can be a part of a meal or serve as a festive appetizer, fitting well within the high-protein, low-carb framework of the carnivore diet.

Loaded Scrambled Eggs

Introduction: Loaded scrambled eggs are a versatile and hearty dish that can be eaten at any meal. Packed with proteins and healthy fats, this dish is meant to keep you satiated and energized throughout your day.

Ingredients:

4 large eggs

1/4 cup milk or cream (optional for creaminess)

1/2 cup cooked and crumbled bacon or sausage

1/4 cup diced bell peppers

1/4 cup shredded cheese (cheddar or your choice)

Salt and pepper to taste

1 tablespoon butter or oil

Five minutes to get ready.

Cooking Time: 10 minutes

15 minutes all together

Instructions:

Prep Ingredients: Heat butter or oil in a pan over medium heat. Add the bell peppers and cook until softened.

Cook Eggs: In a bowl, mix the eggs with milk, salt, and pepper. Pour over the bell peppers in the pan, stirring gently.

Add Fillings: Add the cooked bacon or sausage and cheese. Continue to cook, stirring until the eggs are softly set.

Serve: Serve the scrambled eggs hot, garnished with extra cheese or herbs if desired.

Nutritional Benefits: This dish is a great source of high-quality protein, important for muscle repair and growth, while the added vegetables provide vitamins and fiber.

Dietary Importance: Loaded Scrambled Eggs are a perfect example of a flexible and nutritious meal that can adapt to various dietary needs, giving a strong start to the day or a robust, satisfying lunch.

Ground Beef Stroganoff

Introduction: Ground Beef Stroganoff is a comforting and creamy food that combines simple ingredients to create a rich and flavorful experience, perfect for a family dinner.

Ingredients:

1 pound ground beef

1 onion, chopped

2 cloves garlic, minced

1 cup mushrooms, sliced

1 cup beef broth

1 cup sour cream

2 tablespoons Worcestershire sauce

Salt and pepper to taste

2 tablespoons oil

Fresh parsley, chopped (for garnish)

Preparation Time: 10 minutes

Cooking Time: 20 minutes

Total Time: 30 minutes

Instructions:

Cook Beef: In a pan, heat oil over medium heat. Add the ground beef, onion, and garlic. Cook until the beef is cooked.

Add Mushrooms: Add mushrooms and cook until they are soft.

Simmer: Stir in beef broth and Worcestershire sauce. Bring to a boil and let cook for about 10 minutes until slightly thickened.

Add Sour Cream: Remove from heat and stir in sour cream. Season with salt and pepper.

Serve: Garnish with fresh parsley and serve over noodles or an acceptable substitute for a low-carb option.

Nutritional Benefits:

Rich in protein and iron from the beef, this dish also offers the benefits of sour cream, which includes calcium and additional proteins.

Dietary Importance: Ground Beef Stroganoff is a hearty meal that can provide comfort and happiness, making it easier to stick to dietary goals without feeling deprived.

Creamy Baked Egg Custard

Introduction: Creamy Baked Egg Custard is a simple yet elegant dessert that offers a smooth, comforting texture and a rich taste, perfect for filling sweet cravings healthily.

Ingredients

4 eggs

2 cups milk or cream

1/4 cup sweetener (optional, adjust to diet tastes)

1 teaspoon vanilla extract (optional)

Nutmeg for sprinkling

Preparation Time: 10 minutes

Cooking Time: 45 minutes

Total Time: 55 minutes

Instructions:

Preheat Oven: Preheat your oven to 350°F (175°C).

Mix Ingredients: In a bowl, whisk together eggs, milk, sugar, and vanilla extract until smooth.

Prepare Ramekins: Pour the mixture into ramekins or a baking dish. Sprinkle with nutmeg.

Bake in a Water Bath: Place the ramekins in a baking pan and add hot water to the pan to come halfway up the sides of the ramekins. Bake for 45 minutes, or until set.

Serve: Let cool slightly before serving, or chill in the refrigerator. The custard can be enjoyed warm or cold, making it a versatile dessert option.

Nutritional Benefits: Egg custard is rich in proteins and important nutrients, including calcium and vitamins from the milk or cream. If you're using a sweetener, picking a healthier option can also help maintain blood sugar levels.

Dietary Importance: Creamy Baked Egg Custard is a lovely way to enjoy a dessert that feels indulgent while still adhering to dietary rules that focus on high protein and controlled carbohydrate intake. It can be a delightful treat for those on a ketogenic or low-carb diet, giving a satisfying conclusion to a meal without the guilt often associated with sweets.

Chapter6:Lunch Recipes

Fish Stock Recipe

Introduction: Fish stock is a culinary staple that serves as a rich, flavorful base for various meals such as soups, stews, and sauces. Packed with nutrients, it's especially valued for its high mineral content, including iodine and calcium, which are essential for thyroid function and bone health.

Ingredients

2 pounds fish bones and heads (preferably white fish, cleaned and lungs removed)
1 onion, quartered
2 carrots, chopped; 2 celery stalks, chopped; 1 bay leaf
A few leaves of fresh parsley
1 teaspoon whole peppercorns
8 cups water
Preparation Time: 10 minutes
Cooking Time: 1 hour
Total Time: 1 hour, 10 minutes

Instructions:

Prepare the Ingredients: Rinse the fish bones and heads thoroughly to clear impurities.
Combine Ingredients: In a large pot, add all ingredients and cover with water.
Simmer Gently: Bring to a boil, then reduce to a low simmer. Skim any foam that forms on the top.
Cook: Allow simmering slowly for 1 hour to extract flavors and nutrients.
Strain: Strain the stock through a fine sieve, removing the solids.
Cool and Store: Allow the stock to cool before keeping it in the refrigerator or freezing it for later use.
Health Benefits: Fish stock is rich in collagen, which supports joint health and skin elasticity. It's also a good source of iodine, supporting thyroid health.

Dietary Importance: As a base for numerous recipes, fish stock adds depth and nutrition, improving the health benefits of dishes it's used in, especially for those focusing on a nutrient-dense diet.

Pot Steak Soup

Introduction: Pot Steak Soup is a robust, nutrient-packed meal that combines tender beef with hearty veggies in a flavorful broth, perfect for nourishing the body on a cold day.

Ingredients

1 pound beef steak, cubed 1 onion, chopped 2 carrots, sliced 2 celery stalks, sliced 2 potatoes, cubed 4 cups beef broth, 1 teaspoon dried thyme
Salt and pepper to taste
2 tablespoons olive oil
Preparation Time: 15 minutes
Cooking Time: 1 hour
Total Time: 1 hour 15 minutes

Instructions:

Brown the Beef: In a big pot, heat olive oil over medium heat. Add the meat and brown on all sides.
Add Vegetables: Add onion, carrots, and celery, cooking until cooked.
Simmer: Add potatoes, beef broth, thyme, salt, and pepper. Bring to a boil, then reduce to a simmer for about 1 hour until the beef is soft.
Serve: Adjust salt and serve hot.
Health Benefits: This soup offers a great source of protein, essential amino acids from beef, and vitamins and minerals from vegetables, supporting general health and well-being.

Dietary Importance: Pot Steak Soup provides a balanced meal with proteins, veggies, and a flavorful broth, making it ideal for a healthy diet.

Whole Grilled Chicken

Introduction: Grilling a whole chicken ensures a meal that is not only delicious with a crispy exterior and juicy interior but also nutritionally beneficial, giving a substantial amount of lean protein.

Ingedients:

1 whole chicken (about 4-5 pounds), giblets removed
2 tablespoons olive oil
1 lemon, split
4 garlic cloves, minced
1 tablespoon fresh rosemary, chopped (or 1 teaspoon dried)
Salt and pepper to taste
Preparation Time: 15 minutes (plus extra marinating time)
Cooking Time: 1 hour to 1 hour 30 minutes
Total Time: About 1 hour 45 minutes

Instructions:

Prepare the Chicken: Pat the chicken dry. Rub with olive oil, garlic, rosemary, and season inside and out with salt and pepper.
Preheat the Grill: Heat your grill to medium-high (about 375°F).
Grill the Chicken: Place the chicken breast-side up on the grill. Cover and grill, keeping a consistent temperature, until the internal temperature reaches 165°F.
Rest and Serve: Let the chicken rest for 10 minutes before slicing. Serve with lemon pieces.

Health Benefits: Whole grilled chicken is an excellent source of high-quality protein, which is necessary for muscle repair and immune function. It also offers important B vitamins.

Dietary Importance: This dish is perfect for those seeking a high-protein meal choice that is both filling and flavorful, supporting an active and health-focused lifestyle.

Keto Steak Nuggets
Introduction: Keto Steak Nuggets offer a delicious, bite-sized way to enjoy steak without the carbs. Perfect for snacks or a main dish, these nuggets are rich in proteins and fats, matching with ketogenic dietary needs.

Ingredients

1 pound sirloin steak, trimmed and cut into small cubes
1/2 cup almond flour
1 teaspoon garlic powder
1 teaspoon onion powder
1/2 teaspoon paprika
Salt and pepper to taste
2 large eggs, beaten
2 tablespoons olive oil
Preparation Time: 15 minutes
Cooking Time: 10 minutes

Total Time: 25 minutes

Instructions:

Season the Steak: In a bowl, mix almond flour, garlic powder, onion powder, paprika, salt, and pepper. Dip each steak cube into the beaten eggs, then roll in the almond flour mixture.
Cook: Heat olive oil in a pan over medium heat. Add steak nuggets and cook for about 2-3 minutes per side, or until golden and cooked to your taste.
Serve: Serve hot, with your favorite low-carb dipping sauce.
Nutritional Benefits: Steak is a great source of high-quality protein and fats, necessary for muscle maintenance and overall health. Almond flour offers a low-carb alternative to traditional breading, keeping this dish keto-friendly.

Dietary Importance: These steak nuggets are a satisfying, protein-rich snack or meal that fits perfectly into a ketogenic lifestyle, helping to keep ketosis.

Cheesy Air Fryer Meatballs

Introduction: Cheesy Air Fryer Meatballs are a quick and delicious way to enjoy a keto-friendly version of a classic dish. These meatballs are loaded with cheese and seasoned to perfection, ideal for a cozy meal.

Ingredients

1 pound ground beef (85% lean)
1/2 cup grated Parmesan cheese
1/4 cup mozzarella cheese, chopped into small pieces
1 large egg
2 tablespoons thick cream
1 teaspoon Italian sauce
Salt and pepper to taste. Preparation Time: 10 minutes
Cooking Time: 15 minutes
Total Time: 25 minutes

Instructions:

Mix Ingredients: In a bowl, mix ground beef, Parmesan, mozzarella, egg, heavy cream, Italian seasoning, salt, and pepper. Mix until well mixed.
Form Meatballs: Shape the mixture into small balls, about the size of a golf ball.
Air Fry: Place the meatballs in the air fryer basket, ensuring they do not touch. Cook at 400°F for about 15 minutes, or until browned and cooked through.
Serve: Serve hot, topped with more Parmesan if wanted.
Health Benefits: These meatballs are rich in protein and fats, with cheese adding extra calcium and fatty acids, making them a filling, satisfying part of a ketogenic diet.

Dietary Importance: Perfect for meal prep or a family dinner, these meatballs offer a comforting, keto-friendly option that supports your dietary goals without sacrificing taste.

Keto Taco Pie

Introduction: Keto Taco Pie puts a low-carb take on taco night. This savory pie uses a keto-friendly crust and a flavorful, spiced beef filling, topped with cheese and optional low-carb veggies.

Ingredients

For the crust:
1 1/2 cups almond flour
1/4 cup coconut flour
1/4 cup cold butter, cubed, 1 egg
1/2 teaspoon salt
For the filling:
1 pound ground beef
1/2 onion, chopped

1 packet taco spice (or homemade keto-friendly seasoning)
1 cup shredded cheddar cheese
Optional toppings: cut tomatoes, sliced olives, chopped lettuce
Preparation Time: 20 minutes
Cooking Time: 20 minutes
Total Time: 40 minutes

Instructions:

Prepare the Crust: In a food processor, blend almond flour, coconut flour, butter, egg, and salt until the mixture forms a dough. Press into a pie dish to form a top.
Cook the Filling: In a pan, cook the ground beef and onion until the beef is browned. Drain the extra fat. Stir in the taco sauce.
Assemble the pie: Spoon the meat mixture into the crust. Top with shredded cheese.
Bake: Bake at 350°F for 20 minutes, or until the sides are golden and the cheese is bubbly.
Add Toppings: After baking, add any preferred toppings, like tomatoes, olives, and lettuce.
Serve: Serve warm.
Health Benefits: This taco pie provides a high amount of protein and fats, with the almond and coconut flours providing a low-carb, fiber-rich alternative to traditional crusts.

Dietary Importance: Keto Taco Pie is a creative, delicious dish that allows you to enjoy the flavors of tacos on a ketogenic diet, helping to keep carb intake low while still indulging in your favorite flavors.

Braised Beef Heart with Bone Marrow

Introduction: Braising beef hearts with bone marrow is an excellent way to add nutrient-dense organ meats into your diet. This dish is rich in iron, zinc, and various B vitamins, which are necessary for energy metabolism and overall health.

Ingredients

1 cow heart (about 2-3 pounds), trimmed and cubed
2 bone marrow bones
2 onions, chopped 2 carrots, chopped 2 celery stalks, chopped 4 cloves garlic, minced
2 cups beef broth
1 cup red wine (optional)
2 tablespoons tomato sauce
2 bay leaves
Salt and pepper to taste
2 tablespoons olive oil
Preparation Time: 20 minutes
Cooking Time: 3 hours
Total Time: 3 hours, 20 minutes

Instructions:

Prepare the ingredients: Preheat the oven to 300°F (150°C). Heat olive oil in a large oven-safe pot over medium-high heat. Season beef heart cubes with salt and pepper.
Sear the Meat: Sear the beef heart cubes in batches until cooked on all sides. Remove it and set it aside.
Sauté Vegetables: In the same pot, add onions, carrots, celery, and garlic. Cook until softened.
Deglaze: Pour in red wine (if using) and pick up any browned bits from the bottom of the pot.
Add Liquids and Meat: Stir in tomato paste and beef stock. Return the meat heart and add bone marrow bones to the pot. Add bay leaves.
Braise: Cover and move to the oven. Braise for about 3 hours or until the meat is soft.
Serve: Remove the bay leaves and bone marrow bones. Serve the beef heart with some marrow spread on crusty bread, if requested.

Health Benefits: Beef heart is an excellent source of lean protein and important nutrients like iron and coenzyme Q10, crucial for cardiovascular health. Bone marrow is rich in fat and helps support immune function and bone health.

Dietary Importance: This dish is particularly helpful for those looking to maximize nutrient intake from natural sources. It's a filling, warming meal that supports a nutrient-focused diet.

Organ Meat Pie

Introduction:Organ Meat Pie combines different organ meats in a savory pastry, providing a powerhouse of nutrients. This dish is especially rich in iron, vitamin A, and important amino acids.

Ingredients: 1 pound mixed organ meats (liver, kidney, heart), finely chopped 1 onion, diced
1/2 pound bacon, chopped; 2 cloves garlic, minced
1 teaspoon thyme
1 teaspoon sage
1/2 cup beef broth
Salt and pepper to taste
Pastry dough (enough to line and cover a pie dish)
Preparation Time: 30 minutes
Cooking Time: 1 hour
Total Time: 1 hour, 30 minutes
Instructions:
Preheat the Oven: Preheat your oven to 375°F (190°C).
Cook the Filling: In a pan, cook bacon until crispy. Add onions, garlic, and organ meats. Cook until the foods are browned.
Add Herbs and Broth: Add thyme, sage, and beef broth. Simmer until the liquid is mostly absorbed. Season with salt and pepper.
Assemble the Pie: Line a pie dish with pastry dough. Add the meat combination. Cover with another layer of dough and seal the sides.
Bake: Bake in the prepared oven for about 45 minutes or until the pastry is golden brown.

Serve: Let cool slightly before serving.

Health Benefits: Organ meats are some of the most nutrient-dense foods available, rich in vitamins and minerals that support liver health and brain function.

Dietary Importance: This pie is an excellent way to incorporate a variety of organ meats into your diet, offering a delightful blend of flavors and a boost of important nutrients

.

Protein Pancakes

Introduction: Protein pancakes are a fantastic breakfast choice for those looking to increase their protein intake without sacrificing flavor. Ideal for a post-workout meal or a filling breakfast that keeps you full for hours.
Things used:
1 cup oat flour
1/2 cup protein powder (your pick of flavor)
1 teaspoon baking powder
2 eggs
1 cup Greek yogurt
1/4 cup milk or water
1 tablespoon honey or sweetener of choice
Butter or oil for cooking
Preparation Time: 10 minutes Cooking Time: 10 minutes
Total Time: 20 minutes

Instructions:

Mix Dry Ingredients: In a large bowl, mix oat flour, protein powder, and baking powder.
Combine Wet Ingredients: In another bowl, mix together eggs, Greek yogurt, milk (or water), and honey or sweetener.
Make the batter: Add the wet ingredients to the dry ingredients and stir until just mixed. Let the batter sit for a few minutes to thicken slightly.

Cook the pancakes: Heat a non-stick pan or griddle over medium heat and brush with a small amount of butter or oil. Pour about 1/4 cup of batter for each pancake. Cook until bubbles form on the top, then flip and cook for another 1-2 minutes on the other side until golden brown.

Serve: Serve hot with your choice of toppings, such as fresh berries, yogurt, or sugar-free cream.

Health Benefits: Protein pancakes are a great source of high-quality protein from both the protein powder and Greek yogurt, which helps in muscle repair and satiety. They also offer a good mix of carbohydrates and fats, making them an ideal meal for energy sustenance throughout the day.

Dietary Importance: These pancakes are perfect for those on a fitness or health journey, providing a balanced and satisfying meal that supports muscle health and energy levels without spiking blood sugar. They are also versatile, allowing you to add various flavors and toppings to fit your taste preferences.

Easy Airfryer Carnivore Meatballs Introduction: Enjoy an easy, delicious high-protein dish with these Easy Airfryer Carnivore Meatballs. Perfect for a quick meal or a snack, these meatballs are made exclusively from animal products, aligning with the carnivore diet theory.

Ingredients

1 pound chopped beef (or a mix of beef and pork)
1 egg
Salt and pepper to taste. Preparation Time: 10 minutes
Cooking Time: 10 minutes
Total Time: 20 minutes

Instructions:

Mix Ingredients: In a bowl, mix the ground meat, egg, and a generous amount of salt and pepper. Mix until well mixed.

Form Meatballs: Roll the dough into small balls, about the size of a golf ball.

Air Fry: Place the meatballs in the air fryer basket. Set the air fryer to 400°F and cook for about 10 minutes, or until the meatballs are browned and cooked through.

Serve: Serve hot, with a side of your choice or enjoy them by themselves for a pure carnivore meal.
Health Benefits: These meatballs are rich in protein and fats, important for muscle repair and energy. They are low in carbohydrates, making them ideal for maintaining ketosis if you're also following a ketogenic method.

Dietary Importance: This recipe is great for those strictly adhering to a carnivore diet, focusing on simplicity and high nutrient density without any fillers or plant-based ingredients.

Carnivore Beef Liver Pancakes

Introduction: Carnivore Beef Liver Pancakes blend the nutritional powerhouse of beef liver with the familiar form of pancakes, offering a meal rich in vitamins, especially vitamin A and iron, which are crucial for vision, skin health, and oxygen transport.

Ingredients

1/2 pound cow liver, finely chopped or pureed
2 eggs
Salt to taste Preparation Time: 15 minutes
Cooking Time: 5 minutes per batch
Total Time: 25 minutes

Instructions:

Prepare Liver: Puree the beef liver in a food processor until smooth.
Make Batter: Mix the liver mush with eggs and salt in a bowl.
Cook Pancakes: Heat a pan over medium heat and lightly grease it. Pour small amounts of batter into the pan to make pancakes. Cook for 2-3 minutes per side, or until hard and cooked through.
Serve: Serve warm, possibly with butter or a carnivore-friendly sauce.

Health Benefits: Beef liver is one of the most nutrient-dense foods you can eat, high in vitamin A, iron, and B vitamins.

Dietary Importance: These pancakes are an inventive way to add organ meats into your diet, which can sometimes be a challenge on a carnivore diet.

Meat Lovers Carnivore Pizza

Introduction: Meat Lovers Carnivore Pizza is a zero-carb take on traditional pizza, using ground meat as a base instead of dough, topped with different meats and cheese.

Ingredients

2 pounds ground chicken (for the crust)
1 cup grated Parmesan cheese (for sealing the crust)
1 egg (to help make the crust)
1/2 pound cooked bacon, chopped 1/2 pound ground beef, cooked
1/2 pound sausage, cooked and crumbled
1 cup mozzarella cheese, shredded
Salt and spices to taste
Preparation Time: 20 minutes
Cooking Time: 20 minutes
Total Time: 40 minutes

Instructions:

Make the Crust: Combine ground chicken, Parmesan cheese, egg, and spices. Press the mixture onto a parchment-lined baking sheet, making a thin, even layer.
Pre-Bake the Crust: Bake at 400°F for 10 minutes in a preheated oven, or until the top is firm and beginning to brown.
Add Toppings: Remove the bread from the oven, top with cooked meats and sprinkle with mozzarella cheese.
Bake: Return to the oven and bake for another 10 minutes or until the cheese is bubbly and slightly golden.

Serve: Let cool for a few minutes before slicing and serving.

Health Benefits: This pizza is extremely high in protein and fats, supporting muscle maintenance and providing a high amount of satiety, with minimal carbs.

Dietary Importance: Meat Lovers Carnivore Pizza allows you to enjoy the flavors of a traditional pizza while staying true to the principles of a carnivore diet, making it a satisfying and enjoyable part of your meal plan.

Introduction: Pizza Carnivore Steak Nuggets combine the flavors of pizza with the protein-packed goodness of steak, making them a delightful treat that sticks to a carnivore diet. These nuggets are great as a snack or part of a meal, offering a unique twist on traditional meat dishes.

Ingredients

1 pound sirloin or ribeye steak, cut into bite-sized cubes
1/2 cup grated Parmesan cheese
1 tablespoon Italian sauce
1 teaspoon garlic powder
1 teaspoon onion powder
Salt and pepper to taste
2 eggs, beaten
1 cup pork rind bits
Preparation Time: 15 minutes
Cooking Time: 10 minutes
Total Time: 25 minutes

Instructions:

Season the Steak: In a bowl, mix Parmesan cheese, Italian seasoning, garlic powder, onion powder, salt, and pepper. Toss the steak cubes in this seasoning mix until well coated.

Dip in Eggs: Dip each seasoned steak cube into the beaten eggs, then coat in pork rind crumbs.

Cook: Arrange the nuggets in a single layer in your air fryer basket. Cook at 400°F for about 10 minutes or until the bits are golden brown and cooked through.

Serve: Serve hot with a side of carnivore-friendly marinara sauce if requested.

Health Benefits: Steak provides high-quality protein and important nutrients like iron and zinc, which are crucial for muscle growth and immune function. The use of pork rinds instead of bread crumbs keeps the meal low in carbs and high in satisfying fats.

Dietary Importance: These steak nuggets are an excellent way to enjoy the savory flavors of pizza without straying from a strict carnivore diet, making them a perfect, guilt-free indulgence.

Hidden Liver Meat Muffins

Introduction: Hidden Liver Meat Muffins cleverly combine liver into a palatable form, enriching your diet with one of nature's most nutrient-dense foods. This dish is an excellent way to consume important vitamins and minerals from organ meats without the overwhelming liver taste.

Ingredients

1 pound ground beef
1/2 pound liver (beef or chicken), finely minced or pureed
2 eggs
1 teaspoon salt
1/2 teaspoon black pepper
Optional: herbs and spices for extra flavor
Preparation Time: 20 minutes
Cooking Time: 25 minutes
Total Time: 45 minutes

Instructions:

Preheat Oven: Preheat your oven to 375°F (190°C) and grease a muffin pan.
Mix Ingredients: In a large bowl, mix ground beef, minced liver, eggs, salt, pepper, and any optional herbs and spices. Mix thoroughly.
Fill Muffin Tin: Spoon the meat mixture into the prepared muffin tin, filling each cup about three-quarters full.
Bake: Bake in the prepared oven for 25 minutes or until the meat muffins are cooked through.
Serve: Let cool slightly before taking from the tin. Serve warm.

Health Benefits: Liver is exceptionally rich in vitamin A, iron, and B vitamins, making it great for eyes, skin health, and energy production. Combining it with ground beef improves the protein content, making these muffins both nutritious and filling.

Dietary Importance: Introducing organ meats like liver into your diet can greatly increase your intake of crucial micronutrients. These meat muffins make it easy and fun to get these benefits.

Carnivore Scotch Egg

Introduction: Carnivore Scotch Eggs wrap hard-boiled eggs in a delicious layer of seasoned ground meat, giving a portable and tasty option that fits well within a carnivore diet. They're perfect for breakfast, snacks, or part of a meal.

Ingredients

6 big eggs, hard-boiled
1 pound ground pork or your choice of meat
1 teaspoon salt
1/2 teaspoon black pepper
Optional: herbs and spices to taste
Preparation Time: 20 minutes
Cooking Time: 25 minutes

Total Time: 45 minutes

Instructions:

Preheat Oven: Preheat your oven to 400°F (200°C).
Prepare Eggs: Peel the hard-boiled eggs.
Season the Meat: In a bowl, mix the ground meat with salt, pepper, and any extra herbs and spices.
Wrap the Eggs: Divide the meat mixture into six pieces. Flatten each piece and wrap it around a hard-boiled egg, making sure the egg is completely enclosed.
Bake: Place the meat-wrapped eggs on a baking sheet and bake for 25 minutes or until the meat is fully cooked.
Serve: Serve the Scotch eggs warm or allow them to cool and enjoy them as a cold snack.
Health Benefits: This dish is high in protein and essential fats, giving sustained energy and aiding in muscle repair. The eggs are a great source of choline, which benefits brain health.

Dietary Importance: Carnivore Scotch Eggs are an excellent meal-prep choice for those following a carnivore diet, offering convenience and nutritional density.

Chicken Wings with Aji Verde

Introduction: Chicken Wings with Aji Verde offer a delightful twist on a standard favorite. This dish combines crispy, juicy chicken wings with a vibrant and spicy Peruvian green sauce, making it a perfect choice for parties or a flavorful family meal.

Ingredients

2 pounds chicken wings, tips removed and split at the joint

2 tablespoons olive oil
Salt and pepper to taste
For the Aji Verde:
1 bunch cilantro, leaves and soft stems
2 jalapeños, seeds and chopped
2 cloves garlic
Juice of 1 lime
1/2 cup mayonnaise
Salt to taste
Preparation Time: 20 minutes
Cooking Time: 45 minutes
Total Time: 1 hour 5 minutes

Instructions:

Preheat Oven: Preheat your oven to 400°F (200°C).
Prepare Wings: Toss chicken wings with olive oil, salt, and pepper. Arrange them in a single layer on a baking sheet.
Bake Wings: Bake for 45 minutes or until the flesh is crisp and golden.
Make Aji Verde: While the wings are baking, mix cilantro, jalapeños, garlic, lime juice, and mayonnaise in a blender. Blend until smooth. Season with salt to taste.
Serve: Once the wings are done, allow them to cool slightly, then toss them with the Aji Verde sauce or serve the sauce on the side for dipping.

Health Benefits: Chicken wings are a good source of protein, while the Aji Verde sauce adds a healthy dose of vitamins A and C from the cilantro and jalapeños, which are great for immune support and general well-being.

Dietary Importance: This dish is a fun and tasty way to enjoy a protein-rich meal that can be adapted to fit a keto or low-carb diet, making it flexible and enjoyable for many dietary preferences

Introduction: Meaty Calzones are stuffed with a hearty mix of meats and cheese, wrapped in a golden-brown dough. Perfect for a satisfying meal, these calzones can be made with different fillings to suit your taste.

Ingredients

Pizza dough (baked or store-bought)
1/2 pound ground beef, cooked and drained
1/2 pound Italian sausage, cooked and crumbled
1 cup mozzarella cheese, shredded
1/2 cup ricotta cheese
1/4 cup Parmesan cheese, grated
1/2 cup pizza sauce
1 egg, beaten for egg wash
Preparation Time: 30 minutes
Cooking Time: 20 minutes
Total Time: 50 minutes

Instructions:

Preheat the oven: Preheat your oven to 375°F (190°C).
Prepare Fillings: In a bowl, mix cooked ground beef, sausage, mozzarella, ricotta, and Parmesan cheeses.
Assemble Calzones: Divide the pizza dough into 4 pieces. Roll each piece into a circle. Spoon the meat and cheese mixture onto one half of each circle, leaving a space at the edge. Spoon a little pizza sauce over the filling. Fold the dough over to cover the filling, and crimp the sides to seal.
Apply Egg Wash: Brush the top of each calzone with beaten egg.
Bake: Bake in the prepared oven for about 20 minutes or until golden brown.
Serve: Serve hot, with extra pizza sauce for dipping if wanted.

Health Benefits: Meaty Calzones are rich in protein from the range of meats and cheeses, supporting muscle maintenance and growth. They also offer calcium from the cheese, important for bone health.

Dietary Importance: Calzones provide a filling and customizable meal option, perfect for meal prepping or a family dinner. Adjusting the fillings can cater to different dietary needs and tastes.

Slow Cooker Hamburger Soup

Introduction: Slow Cooker Hamburger Soup is a hearty, comforting dish that's great for busy days. Packed with vegetables, beef, and broth, it's both nutritious and satisfying, providing a warm meal at the end of the day.

Ingredients

1 pound ground beef, cooked and drained
3 carrots, peeled and diced
3 celery stalks, diced 1 onion, diced 2 potatoes, peeled and cubed 1 can (28 oz) diced tomatoes
4 cups beef broth, 2 teaspoons dried basil
Salt and pepper to taste
Preparation Time: 15 minutes
Cooking Time: 8 hours on low Total Time: 8 hours, 15 minutes

Instructions:

Prepare Ingredients: Place all ingredients in a slow cooker.
Cook: Set the slow cooker to low and cook for about 8 hours, or until the veggies are tender.
Season: Adjust flavor with salt and pepper before serving.
Serve: Serve hot, garnished with fresh parsley if wanted.

Health Benefits: This soup is a great source of protein, carbohydrates, vitamins, and minerals. It's ideal for a balanced diet, giving important nutrients needed for daily activities and overall health.

Dietary Importance: Hamburger Soup is especially beneficial for those wanting a nutritious, low-effort meal that can be prepared in advance and enjoyed throughout the week, fitting well into a busy lifestyle while supporting dietary goals.

Baguettes (Easy 5 Ingredients)

Introduction: Homemade baguettes bring the charm of French bakeries into your home. This simple recipe uses only five basic ingredients to make crispy, fluffy baguettes that are perfect for sandwiches, soups, or to enjoy with butter.

Ingredients

4 cups all-purpose flour
1 teaspoon salt 1 teaspoon sugar 1 packet (2 1/4 teaspoons) active dry yeast
1 1/2 cups warm water (about 110°F)
Preparation Time: 20 minutes + 2 hours for rising
Cooking Time: 25 minutes
Total Time: About 2 hours 45 minutes

Instructions:

Prepare the Dough: In a large bowl, mix flour, salt, and sugar. In a small bowl, dissolve the yeast in warm water and let sit for 5 minutes until foamy. Add the yeast mixture to the flour and stir until a dough forms.
Knead the Dough: Turn the dough onto a floured surface and knead for about 10 minutes until smooth and springy.
First Rise: Place the dough in an oiled bowl, cover with a damp cloth, and let rise in a warm place for about 1.5 hours, or until doubled in size.
Shape and Second Rise: Punch down the dough and split it into two pieces. Roll each piece into a long, thin loaf. Place on a baking sheet, cover lightly, and let rise for another 30 minutes.

Bake: Preheat your oven to 450°F (230°C). Make several vertical slashes on top of each loaf with a sharp knife. Bake for 25 minutes, or until golden brown and hollow sounding when hit.

Serve: Let the baguettes cool slightly before slicing. Serve warm or at room temperature.

Health Benefits: Baguettes provide carbohydrates for energy, and if made with whole wheat flour, can also offer fiber and extra nutrients.

Dietary Importance: While easy, baking your own bread can be a rewarding experience that adds a fresh, wholesome element to your meals, allowing for control over ingredients and avoiding preservatives found in store-bought bread.

Bacon wrapped scallops

Introduction: Bacon scallops are a luxurious appetizer great for impressing guests or treating yourself. This dish combines the sweetness of scallops with the savory richness of bacon, giving a mouthwatering flavor contrast.

Ingredients

12 large sea scallops
12 slices of bacon
1 tablespoon olive oil
Salt and pepper to taste
Toothpicks
Preparation Time: 15 minutes
Cooking Time: 15 minutes
Total Time: 30 minutes

Instructions:

Prepare the Scallops: Pat the scallops dry with paper towels and season with salt and pepper.

Wrap with Bacon: Wrap each scallop with a piece of bacon and secure with a toothpick.

Cook: Heat olive oil in a big skillet over medium-high heat. Add the bacon-wrapped scallops and cook, turning occasionally, until the bacon is crispy and the scallops are opaque, about 15 minutes.

Serve: Remove from heat and place on a paper towel-lined plate to absorb extra grease. Serve hot, garnished with fresh herbs if wanted.

Health Benefits: Scallops are a great source of protein and provide essential vitamins and minerals, including B12 and zinc. Bacon adds a delightful taste, though it should be enjoyed in moderation due to its fat content.

Dietary Importance: This dish is a great example of how indulgent foods can be introduced into a balanced diet, providing a source of high-quality protein while satisfying cravings for something rich and savory.

Carnivore Stroganoff

Introduction: This dish takes a traditional Russian dish and changes it so that it's all about meat. It uses only animal-based ingredients to make a creamy, filling meal that is both comforting and follows the rules for a carnivore's diet.

Ingredients:

2 pounds of beef sirloin, cut into thin slices
One cup of sour cream and two cups of beef soup
Add salt and pepper to taste.
2 sticks of butter
Ten minutes to get ready.
Twenty minutes of cooking time
30 minutes all together

Instructions

Melt the butter over medium-high heat in a big skillet. Add the beef and brown it. Add the meat slices and sear until browned on all sides. Season with salt and pepper.
Simmer: Reduce heat to medium. Add beef broth to the pan and let it simmer for about 10 minutes, or until the beef is tender.
Add Sour Cream: Reduce the heat to low and stir in sour cream. Cook softly, just until the sauce is heated through. Avoid boiling to avoid curdling.
Serve: Serve warm. This dish can be enjoyed as is for a pure carnivore meal or over a bed of buttered zucchini noodles if wanted.

Health Benefits: Beef is a great source of high-quality protein and provides important nutrients like iron and B vitamins. Sour cream adds fat for energy and satisfaction.

Dietary Importance: This version of stroganoff is great for those following a carnivore diet, focusing on high-protein and high-fat intake while excluding non-animal ingredients.

Beef Patties with Onion Gravy

Introduction: Beef Patties with Onion Gravy is a hearty and delicious dish that combines juicy beef patties with a rich onion gravy, perfect for a comforting and satisfying dinner.

Ingredients:

1 pound ground beef
1 large onion, sliced
2 cups beef broth
1 tablespoon butter
Salt and pepper to taste Preparation Time: 15 minutes
Cooking Time: 25 minutes
Total Time: 40 minutes

Instructions

Form burgers: Shape the ground beef into 4 burgers. Season with salt and pepper.
Cook Patties: In a pan, melt butter over medium heat. Add the patties and cook until browned on both sides and cooked to your chosen doneness. Remove it and set it aside.
Make Onion Gravy: In the same pan, add the sliced onions. Cook them until they are soft and golden. Pour in the beef broth and bring to a simmer. Let it reduce slightly until it thickens.
Serve: Return the meat patties to the skillet and coat them with the onion gravy. Serve hot.

Health Benefits: This dish provides a good amount of protein, which is necessary for muscle maintenance and growth. Onions add a small amount of vitamins and antioxidants.

Dietary Importance: Beef patties with onion gravy offer a nutrient-rich, satisfying meal that fits well into a diet based on whole, minimally processed foods.

Chicken Liver Pâté

Introduction: Chicken Liver Pâté is a nutrient-dense appetizer or side dish, rich in vitamins and minerals, especially iron and vitamin A, which support immune function and vision.

Ingredients:

1 pound chicken livers, cleaned and chopped
1/2 cup butter, divided 1 onion, chopped 2 cloves garlic, minced
1/4 cup heavy cream
2 tablespoons brandy or cognac (optional)
Add salt and pepper to taste.
Preparation Time: 15 minutes
Cooking Time: 10 minutes
Total Time: 25 minutes + chilling

Instructions:

Cook Livers: In a pan, melt half the butter over medium heat. Add onion and garlic, sauté until translucent. Add chicken livers and cook until they are browned but still slightly pink in the middle.
Blend: Transfer the liver mixture to a food processor. Add heavy cream, brandy (if using), leftover butter, salt, and pepper. Blend until smooth.
Chill: Pour the liquid into a small bowl or ramekin. Cover and chill for at least 2 hours until firm.

Serve: Serve chilled, spread on low-carb crackers or vegetable slices for a full carnivore diet meal.

Health Benefits: Chicken liver is incredibly rich in nutrients, giving high levels of vitamin A, iron, and various B vitamins. These are important for energy, metabolism, and overall health.

Dietary Importance: Chicken liver pâté is an excellent way to introduce organ meats into your diet. They are known for their

Homemade Deli-Style Roast Beef

Introduction: Homemade Deli-Style Roast Beef offers a healthier, preservative-free choice than store-bought options. This recipe allows you to enjoy tender, flavorful roast beef made right in your kitchen, great for sandwiches or as a main meal.

Ingredients

2 pounds beef eye round roast
2 tablespoons olive oil
1 tablespoon kosher salt 2 teaspoons black pepper
1 teaspoon garlic powder
1 teaspoon onion powder
1 teaspoon dried thyme
Ten minutes to get ready.
Cooking Time: 1 hour to 1 hour 30 minutes
Total Time: About 1 hour, 40 minutes + resting time

Instructios:

Preheat the oven: Preheat your oven to 375°F (190°C).

Season the Beef: Rub the beef all over with olive oil. Mix salt, pepper, garlic powder, onion powder, and thyme together, then rub this mixture all over the beef.

Roast: Place the seasoned beef on a rack in a baking pan. Roast in the preheated oven for about 1 to 1.5 hours, or until the internal temperature hits 135°F (57°C) for medium rare.

Rest: Remove the roast from the oven and let it rest for at least 20 minutes before chopping. This helps the juices to redistribute.

Serve: Slice thinly against the grain and serve as requested.

Health Benefits: Roast beef is an excellent source of high-quality protein and iron, which are important for muscle repair and oxygen transport in the blood.

Dietary Importance: Making your own roast beef ensures control over ingredients, avoiding the high sodium and preservatives often found in deli meats, making this a healthier choice for those watching their dietary intake closely.

Keto-Carnivore Black Pudding

Introduction: Keto-Carnivore Black Pudding puts a unique spin on a classic dish, using low-carb ingredients to fit ketogenic and carnivore diets. This dish is rich in iron and protein, making it a savory breakfast or side dish.

Ingredients:

1 pound pork blood 1/2 pound pork fat, finely chopped
1/4 cup pork rinds, ground
1 teaspoon salt
1/2 teaspoon black pepper
1/2 teaspoon dried allspice
Optional: fresh herbs for taste
Preparation Time: 20 minutes
Cooking Time: 1 hour
Total Time: 1 hour, 20 minutes

Instructions:

Mix Ingredients: In a large bowl, mix pork blood, diced pork fat, ground pork rinds, salt, pepper, and allspice (and herbs if using). Mix thoroughly.

Fill Casings: If available, fill sausage casings with the mixture. Alternatively, pour the mixture into a loaf pan.

Cook: If using shells, steam or simmer in water for about 1 hour. If using a loaf pan, bake in a water bath at 325°F (163°C) for 1 hour.

Cool and Serve: Allow to cool completely before slicing. Serve it cold or lightly fried.

Health Benefits: Black pudding is an excellent source of protein and iron, which are important for maintaining energy levels and supporting immune function.

Dietary Importance: This recipe provides a keto-friendly and carnivore-appropriate version of black pudding, ideal for those following strict dietary regimens without sacrificing taste or cultural culinary experiences.

Instant Pot Steak Soup

Introduction: Instant Pot Steak Soup is a hearty, comforting meal that can be made quickly and easily in your Instant Pot. This soup is packed with tender steak, nutritious vegetables, and a flavorful broth, making it a great meal for any day of the week.

Ingredients:

1 pound steak, cubed, 2 tablespoons olive oil
1 onion, chopped 2 carrots, sliced 2 stalks celery, sliced 2 cloves garlic, minced
4 cups beef broth
1 teaspoon dried thyme
Add salt and pepper to taste.
Preparation Time: 15 minutes
Cooking Time: 30 minutes

Total Time: 45 minutes

Instructionss:

Sauté Ingredients: Set your Instant Pot to 'Sauté' mode. Add olive oil, onion, carrots, celery, and garlic. Cook until softened.
Brown the Steak: Add the steak cubes and sauté until browned on all sides.
Add Broth and Seasonings: Pour in beef broth, adding thyme, salt, and pepper.
Pressure Cook: Close the lid and set the Instant Pot to 'Manual' or 'Pressure Cook' mode for 20 minutes.
Release and Serve: After cooking, let the air release naturally for 10 minutes, then manually release any remaining pressure. Stir the soup, fix seasoning if needed, and serve hot.

Health Benefits: This soup offers a great balance of protein, essential fats, and vitamins from the vegetables, giving a well-rounded meal that supports overall health.

Dietary Importance: Steak soup in the Instant Pot is an efficient way to make a nutrient-dense meal that fits into a busy lifestyle, ensuring you get a comforting and healthy dinner on the table quickly.   nutrient content, supporting a robust and nourishing dietary approach.

Osso Bucco Made Easy

Introduction: Traditional Italian food, Osso Bucco, is made with slow-cooked veal shanks that are braised to make a tender, flavorful meal. This easier version still gets the point across and takes less time to make, making it perfect for a special dinner.

Ingredients:

4 calf shanks that are about an inch thick
2 tsp. olive oil, salt, and pepper to taste

1 onion, cut up small
1 carrot, cut up small
1 celery stalk, cut up very small
Two cloves of chopped garlic
1 cup dry white wine
1 cup beef broth
1 can diced tomatoes
1 teaspoon dried thyme
1 bay leaf
Preparation Time: 20 minutes
Cooking Time: 2 hours
Total Time: 2 hours, 20 minutes

Instructions:

Preheat the oven: Preheat your oven to 325°F (163°C).
Season the Veal: Season the veal shanks with salt and pepper.
Brown the Veal: In a large ovenproof pot, heat olive oil over medium-high heat. Brown the veal shanks on all sides and set aside.
Sauté Vegetables: In the same pot, add onion, carrot, celery, and garlic. Sauté until softened.
Deglaze and Simmer: Add white wine to deglaze the pot, picking up any browned bits. Add beef broth, chopped tomatoes, thyme, and bay leaf. Bring to a simmer.
Braise: Return the veal shanks to the pot. Cover and move to the oven. Braise for about 2 hours or until the meat is soft.
Serve: Discard the bay leaf. Serve the veal shanks with the veggie sauce spooned over them.

Health Benefits: Veal is rich in high-quality protein and essential nutrients such as zinc, phosphorus, and B vitamins, especially vitamin B12, which supports nerve health and energy metabolism.

Dietary Importance: Osso Bucco is a nutrient-dense, hearty dish that fits well within a balanced diet, providing substantial nourishment and pleasure.

Introduction: Carnivore Pizza reimagines classic pizza with a meat-based crust and toppings, perfect for those avoiding carbs and sticking to animal-based ingredients.

Ingredients

For the crust:
2 cups ground chicken or turkey
1 egg
Add salt and pepper to taste.
Toppings:
1 cup shredded mozzarella cheese
1/2 cup cooked bacon, chopped
Additional toppings as per diet compliance (e.g., more cheese, small amounts of sauce if allowed)
Preparation Time: 15 minutes
Twenty minutes of cooking time
Total Time: 35 minutes

Ingridients:

Preheat the oven: Preheat your oven to 400°F (204°C).
Prepare Crust: Mix ground chicken with egg, salt, and pepper. Press the mixture onto a lined baking sheet, making a thin, even layer.
Pre-Bake Crust: Bake the crust for 10 minutes, then remove from the oven.
Add Toppings: Sprinkle mozzarella cheese over the bread, add cooked bacon, and any other carnivore-friendly toppings.
Bake: Return to the oven and bake for an additional 10 minutes or until the cheese is melted and bubbly.
Serve: Slice and serve hot.

Health Benefits: The crust made from ground chicken provides a good form of protein, while cheese adds calcium and additional protein, supporting muscle and bone health.

Dietary Importance: Carnivore Pizza allows individuals following a carnivore diet to enjoy a familiar comfort food in a way that fits with their dietary restrictions, ensuring they can indulge in a satisfying meal without compromise.

Pressure Cooker Pork Loin Roast

Introduction: Pressure Cooker Pork Loin Roast is a tender, juicy dish that's quick and easy to make. Cooking in a pressure cooker not only saves time but also preserves the nutrients, making it a healthy choice for a hearty family meal.

Ingredients

2 pounds pork loin roast
2 tablespoons olive oil
1 onion, sliced
4 cloves garlic, minced
1 cup chicken broth
1 tablespoon dried rosemary
1 tablespoon dried thyme
Salt and pepper to taste. Preparation Time: 10 minutes
Cooking Time: 60 minutes
Total Time: 70 minutes

Instructions

Season the Pork: Rub the pork chops with salt, pepper, rosemary, and thyme.
Brown the Pork: Heat olive oil in the pressure cooker on the sauté setting. Add the pork chops and sear on all sides until golden brown.

Add Ingredients: Remove the pork and set away. Add onions and garlic to the cooker and sauté until softened. Place the pork back in the pot and add chicken broth.

Cook: Secure the lid of the pressure cooker and set it to cook under high pressure for 50 minutes.

Natural Release: Let the pressure release gradually after cooking.

Serve: Slice the pork belly and serve with the cooking juices drizzled over the top.

Health Benefits: Pork loin is a lean protein source, important for muscle repair and maintenance. It is also rich in vitamins B6 and B12, which help in energy production and brain health.

Dietary Importance: This method of cooking saves most of the nutrients, providing a healthy meal that can fit into various dietary plans, especially for those needing high-protein meals.

Grilled Bone Marrow with Garlic Parmesan Crust

Introduction: Grilled Bone Marrow with Garlic Parmesan Crust is an indulgent dish, giving rich flavors and a myriad of health benefits. Bone marrow is a delicacy that is rich in nutrients, making this dish not only delicious but also helpful for health.

Ingredients:

4 large beef bones, cut lengthwise (marrow visible)
4 cloves garlic, minced
1/2 cup grated Parmesan cheese
1/4 cup chopped parsley
2 tablespoons olive oil
Salt and pepper to taste Preparation Time: 15 minutes
Cooking Time: 15 minutes
30 minutes all together

Instructions:

Preheat the grill: Preheat your grill to medium-high heat.
Prepare the marrow: Season the bone marrow with salt and pepper. Mix olive oil, garlic, Parmesan, and parsley in a bowl. Spread this mixture over the meat.
fire: Place the bones marrow side up on the fire. Grill for about 15 minutes, or until the marrow is bubbly and the top is golden.
Serve: Serve quickly, scooping out the marrow to spread on toasted bread or enjoy as is.

Health Benefits: Bone marrow is rich in collagen, which is good for skin and joint health, and provides important fatty acids and vitamins.

Dietary Importance: This dish is a luxurious way to add high-quality fats into your diet, which can be beneficial for those following keto or paleo diets.

Herb Roasted Bone Marrow

Introduction: Herb Roasted Bone Marrow is a simple yet exotic meal that serves as a great appetizer or a side dish. The roasting process brings out the flavor of the marrow, while the herbs add a fresh contrast.

Things used:

6 beef marrow bones, cut crosswise
2 tablespoons fresh rosemary, chopped
2 tablespoons fresh thyme, chopped
Salt and ground black pepper
Olive oil
Ten minutes to get ready.
Twenty minutes of cooking time
30 minutes all together

How to Do It:

Preheat the oven: Preheat your oven to 450°F (230°C).

Prepare Bones: Place the bones on a baking sheet, flesh side up. Drizzle with olive oil and season with salt, pepper, rosemary, and thyme.

Roast: Roast in the oven for about 20 minutes, or until the marrow is softened and has started to bubble.

Serve: Serve hot, followed by a sprinkle of sea salt and crusty bread for scooping out the marrow.

Nutritional Benefits: Like grilled bone marrow, this dish is high in collagen and healthy fats, which are vital for maintaining good health and supporting immune function.

Dietary Importance: Herb Roasted Bone Marrow offers a nutrient-dense treat that complements a low-carb, high-fat diet perfectly, making it a favored choice for those on ketogenic or carnivore diets.

Introduction: Mozzarella-Stuffed Meatballs combine the juicy, savory taste of meatballs with a gooey, cheesy center, making them a great dish for family dinners or gatherings. These meatballs can be eaten on their own, with pasta, or in a sub for a delicious meal.

Ingredients

1 pound ground beef
1/2 pound chopped pork
1 cup breadcrumbs
1/4 cup milk
1 egg
Two cloves of chopped garlic
1/2 cup grated Parmesan cheese
1 teaspoon salt
1/2 teaspoon black pepper

1 teaspoon Italian sauce
Small cheese balls (or cubed mozzarella)
2 cups tomato sauce
Preparation Time: 20 minutes
Cooking Time: 30 minutes
Total Time: 50 minutes

Instructions:

Preheat Oven: Preheat your oven to 400°F (200°C).
Mix Ingredients: In a large bowl, mix ground beef, ground pork, breadcrumbs, milk, egg, garlic, Parmesan, salt, pepper, and Italian seasoning. Mix well until evenly mixed.
Form Meatballs: Take a small piece of the meat mixture, flatten it in your hand, place a mozzarella ball in the center, and wrap the meat around the cheese. Roll it into a ball, ensuring the cheese is completely enclosed.
Cook Meatballs: Place the stuffed meatballs on a baking sheet. Bake in the prepared oven for about 20 minutes.
Simmer in Sauce: Heat marinara sauce in a pot. Add the baked meatballs to the sauce and let them boil for about 10 minutes.
Serve: Serve hot with a sprinkling of fresh basil or parsley, if preferred.

Health Benefits: These meatballs are a good source of protein and iron. The combination of meats gives high-quality protein, while the mozzarella offers calcium for bone health.

Dietary Importance: Mozzarella-stuffed meatballs are a comforting and satisfying dish that can be adapted to fit into different dietary needs, including low-carb and ketogenic diets, when served without pasta.

Chicken Taco Soup

Introduction: Chicken Taco Soup is a hearty and delicious dish packed with the robust flavors of a taco in a comforting soup form. It's easy to make and great for a nutritious weeknight meal.

Ingredients:

2 chicken breasts
1 onion, chopped
Two cloves of chopped garlic
1 bell pepper, chopped
1 can black beans, drained and rinsed (optional, skip for keto/paleo diets)
1 can corn, drained (optional, skip for keto/paleo diets)
1 can chopped tomatoes
4 cups chicken broth
2 teaspoons chili sauce
1 teaspoon cumin
Add salt and pepper to taste.
Avocado, sour cream, and chopped cheese for garnish
Ten minutes to get ready.
Cooking Time: 30 minutes
Total Time: 40 minutes

Instructions:

Cook Chicken: In a big pot, add a little oil and cook the chicken breasts until fully cooked. Remove, shred, and set away.

Sauté Vegetables: In the same pot, add onion, garlic, and bell pepper. Cook until soft.

Combine Ingredients: Return the shredded chicken to the pot. Add beans, corn, chopped tomatoes, chicken broth, chili powder, cumin, salt, and pepper.

Simmer: Bring to a boil, then reduce heat and simmer for 20 minutes.

Serve: Ladle the soup into cups and garnish with avocado, sour cream, and shredded cheese.

Health Benefits: This soup is rich in protein from chicken, vitamins and minerals from veggies, and fiber from beans and corn. It's a great meal for energy and nutrient intake.

Dietary Importance: Chicken taco soup is adaptable to different diets by modifying or omitting certain ingredients. It's filling and nutritious, giving a balanced meal with proteins, vitamins, and minerals.

Stream Tartare (Assuming Fresh Fish Tartare)

Introduction: Stream tartare, typically made with fresh, high-quality fish, is a delicate and elegant dish that's great for a sophisticated appetizer or a light meal. It's fresh, zesty, and full of tastes.

Ingredients:

1 pound fresh salmon or trout, finely chopped
1 small onion, minced, 1 tablespoon capers, chopped, 1 tablespoon fresh dill, chopped
Juice of 1 lemon
Salt and black pepper to taste
Olive oil for drizzling
Preparation Time: 15 minutes
Cooking Time: 0 minutes
15 minutes all together

Ingredients:

Prepare Fish: Ensure the fish is fresh and of sushi-grade quality. Finely chop the fish and place it in a mixing bowl.
Mix Ingredients: Add onion, capers, dill, and lemon juice to the chopped fish. Season with salt and pepper.
Chill: Cover the mixture and refrigerate for about 10 minutes to allow the tastes to meld.
Serve: Serve the tartare on small plates or crackers, topped with a bit of olive oil.

Health Benefits: Fresh fish is an excellent source of omega-3 fatty acids, which are important for heart health and cognitive functions. The addition of lemon offers vitamin C, enhancing iron absorption and immune support.

Dietary Importance: Fish tartare is a great choice for those focused on high-quality proteins and heart-healthy fats. It's particularly suitable for diets that prioritize fresh, minimally processed foods.

Introduction: A Perfectly Seared Ribeye Steak is a classic favorite that stands out for its rich taste and tender texture. Using grass-fed beef not only enhances this dish with a superior taste but also with increased nutritional benefits, making it a beloved choice for a special event or a gourmet dinner at home.

Ingredients:

1 grass-fed ribeye steak (about 1-inch thick)
Salt and finely ground black pepper
2 tablespoons olive oil
2 cloves garlic, lightly crushed
2 sprigs fresh thyme or rosemary
2 sticks of butter
Five minutes to get ready.
Cooking Time: 6 to 8 minutes
Total Time: Approximately 15 minutes, including stopping time

Ingredients:

Preheat Pan: Heat a heavy pan (preferably cast iron) over high heat until very hot.
Season Steak: Generously season the steak with salt and pepper on both sides.

Sear Steak: Add olive oil to the hot skillet, then put the steak in the pan. Sear for about 3 minutes per side for medium-rare, or adjust according to your taste.

Add Flavorings: Halfway through cooking, add the garlic, herbs, and butter to the pan. As the butter melts, spoon it over the steak constantly to baste.

Rest the Steak: Remove the steak from the pan and let it rest for at least 5 minutes to allow the juices to spread.

Serve: Slice against the grain and serve quickly.

Health Benefits: Grass-fed beef is richer in omega-3 fatty acids and antioxidants than grain-fed meat. It also provides high-quality protein and important nutrients such as iron and zinc.

Dietary Importance: This dish supports a balanced diet focused on high-quality proteins and healthy fats, which are necessary for muscle maintenance, brain function, and general health.

Succulent Braised Short Ribs

Introduction: Braised Short Ribs are a great comfort food, known for their deep flavors and tender meat that falls off the bone. Slow-cooked in a rich sauce, these ribs are not only delicious but also packed with nutrients.

Ingredients:

4 pounds beef short ribs
Salt and black pepper
2 tablespoons vegetable oil
1 onion, chopped 2 carrots, chopped 2 celery stalks, chopped 2 cups beef broth 1 cup red wine (optional)
2 tablespoons tomato sauce
Fresh herbs (thyme, rosemary)
Preparation Time: 20 minutes
Cooking Time: 3 hours

Total Time: About 3 hours, 20 minutes

Instructions:

Prepare Ribs: Season the short ribs heavily with salt and pepper.
Brown Ribs: In a large Dutch oven or heavy pot, heat oil over medium-high heat. Add the ribs and brown on all sides, then remove and set away.
Sauté Vegetables: In the same pot, add onion, carrots, and celery. Cook until softened.
Deglaze and Simmer: Stir in tomato paste, then add wine (if using) and beef broth. Bring to a boil, scraping up any browned bits from the bottom of the pot.
Braise: Return the ribs to the pot. Add herbs, cover, and move to a 325°F (163°C) oven. Braise for about 2.5 to 3 hours until the meat is very soft.
Serve: Remove the herbs and serve the ribs with the braising stock as a sauce.

Health Benefits: Beef short ribs provide a rich source of protein and vital fatty acids. The vegetables and broth add vitamins and minerals, enhancing the dish's nutritional profile.

Dietary Importance: This meal is excellent for those needing high-energy, nutrient-dense foods, especially in colder months or for healing meals.

Oven-Roasted Bone Marrow

Introduction: Oven-Roasted Bone Marrow is a delicacy rich in taste and nutrients. Often referred to as "nature's butter," bone marrow provides a host of benefits from healthy fats and minerals, making it a prized component in foodie and health-conscious kitchens alike.

Ingredients:

6 beef or chicken marrow bones, cut into 2-inch pieces
Salt and ground black pepper
Fresh parsley, finely chopped (for garnish)

Ten minutes to get ready.
Twenty minutes of cooking time
30 minutes all together

Instructions:

Preheat the oven: Preheat your oven to 450°F (230°C).
Prepare Bones: Place the marrow bones on a baking sheet, marrow side up. Season lightly with salt and pepper.
Roast: Roast in the preheated oven for about 20 minutes, or until the marrow is soft, bubbling, and slightly browned at the sides.
Serve: Sprinkle with chopped parsley and serve quickly with toast points or crusty bread for scooping.

Health Benefits: Bone marrow is rich in collagen, which supports skin, joint, and gut health, and provides important fatty acids for brain function and reducing inflammation.

Dietary Importance: Including bone marrow in your diet can improve your intake of healthy fats and minerals, supporting a balanced and nutrient-rich diet.

Grass-Fed Beef Liver Chips

Introduction: These chips are a unique and healthy way to get the health benefits of liver. These chips are a tasty, crunchy snack that can also be used as a side dish. They are high in important nutrients.

Ingredients:

grass-fed beef liver, cut into thin slices, 1 pound
Half a cup of tapioca starch or arrowroot powder
Add salt and pepper to taste.
Fry-safe cooking oil, like lard or coconut oil
15 minutes to get ready.
Ten minutes of cooking time

25 minutes all together

Instructions:

Prepare the liver by washing the pieces and patting them dry. Season with salt and pepper.
Dust with Starch: Lightly dust the liver slices in arrowroot powder or tapioca starch, shaking off any extra.
Heat Oil: In a big frying pan, heat the cooking oil over medium-high heat.
Fry Liver: Fry the liver slices in batches, being careful not to overcrowd the pan. Cook each side for about 1-2 minutes or until crispy.
Drain: Remove the chips and drain on paper towels.
Serve: Serve hot as a snack or side dish.

Health Benefits: Beef liver is extremely nutrient-dense, providing high amounts of vitamin A, iron, and B vitamins, which are vital for energy metabolism and immune system function.

Dietary Importance: These liver chips are a great way to add organ meats into your diet, especially if you are following a carnivore or paleo diet, providing important nutrients that support overall health.

Grass-Fed Beef Stroganoff

Introduction: Grass-Fed Beef Stroganoff is a creamy, comforting dish made with high-quality beef that not only tastes better but is also richer in omega-3 fatty acids compared to grain-fed meat. This dish blends tender beef with a rich and tangy sour cream sauce.

Ingredients:

2 pounds grass-fed beef sirloin, thinly sliced
2 sticks of butter
1 onion, cut up small
Two cloves of chopped garlic

1 cup mushrooms, sliced
1 cup beef broth
1 cup sour cream
2 teaspoons Dijon mustard
Add salt and pepper to taste.
Fresh parsley, chopped (for garnish)
15 minutes to get ready.
Twenty minutes of cooking time
Total Time: 35 minutes

Ingredients:

Sauté Beef: In a big skillet, melt butter over medium heat. Add the beef and sauté until browned. Remove the beef and set it away.
Cook Vegetables: In the same pan, add onions and garlic. Cook until softened. Add mushrooms and cook until soft.
Combine Ingredients: Return the beef to the skillet. Add beef broth and bring to a simmer. Reduce heat and stir in sour cream and Dijon mustard. Cook gently until warm through but not boiling.
Season: Season with salt and pepper.
Serve: Garnish with fresh parsley and serve over egg noodles or mashed potatoes for a satisfying meal.

Health Benefits: This dish is rich in protein and vital fats, along with being a good source of selenium and zinc, which are important for antioxidant defense and immune health.

Dietary Importance: Beef Stroganoff is perfect for a low-carb, high-protein diet, providing sustained energy and important nutrients while satisfying hunger.

Perfectly Grilled Lamb Chops

Introduction: Perfectly Grilled Lamb Chops are a luxurious and easy meal, known for their rich flavor and tenderness. Lamb is an excellent source of high-quality protein and vital nutrients, making it a favorite for special events or a gourmet weekend dinner.

Ingredients:

8 lamb chops
2 tablespoons olive oil
Two cloves of chopped garlic
1 tablespoon rosemary, chopped
Add salt and pepper to taste.
Preparation Time: 10 minutes (plus soaking time)
Ten minutes of cooking time
Total Time: 20 minutes + marinating time

Intructions:

Marinate Lamb: In a bowl, mix olive oil, garlic, rosemary, salt, and pepper. Coat the lamb chops in the marinade and let sit for at least 30 minutes or up to a few hours in the fridge.
Preheat the grill: Preheat your grill to medium-high heat.
Grill Lamb Chops: Place the lamb chops on the grill and cook for about 3-4 minutes per side for medium-rare, or adjust according to your desired doneness.
Rest: Let the chops rest for a few minutes after cooking.
Serve: Serve quickly, perhaps with a side of grilled vegetables or a fresh salad.

Nutritional Benefits: Lamb is an excellent source of iron, zinc, and B vitamins, especially B12, which is crucial for neurological function and blood formation.

Dietary Importance: Grilled lamb chops provide a nutrient-rich, keto-friendly choice that fits well within a balanced diet, emphasizing protein and essential fats without added carbs.

Introduction: Smokey Bacon-Wrapped Chicken Thighs offer a delightful mix of juicy chicken and crispy bacon, infused with smoky flavors. This dish is perfect for a comforting dinner and is sure to fill your craving for something savory and hearty.

Ingredients:

8 boneless, skinless chicken thighs
16 slices of bacon
1 tablespoon smoked pepper
Salt and black pepper to taste Optional: bbq sauce for brushing
15 minutes to get ready.
Cooking Time: 40 minutes
Total Time: 55 minutes

Ingredients:

Preheat the oven: Preheat your oven to 375°F (190°C).
Season Chicken: Season chicken legs with smoked paprika, salt, and pepper.
Wrap with Bacon: Wrap each leg with two slices of bacon, securing the ends with toothpicks if necessary.
Arrange on Baking Tray: Place the bacon-wrapped legs on a wire rack over a baking sheet to catch drippings.
Bake: Bake in the prepared oven for about 30 minutes. If using, brush with barbecue sauce and bake for an additional 10 minutes until the bacon is crispy and the chicken is thoroughly cooked.
Serve: Let rest for a few minutes before serving to allow the juices to spread.

Nutritional Benefits: Chicken thighs are a great source of protein, while bacon adds a delicious richness. This dish offers essential amino acids and B vitamins.

Dietary Importance: Perfect for low-carb and keto diets, this dish focuses on high protein and fat content, which can help in maintaining muscle mass and promoting satiety.

Carnivore Home Cooked Mac n' Cheese

Introduction: Carnivore Mac n' Cheese is a creative, low-carb take on the classic comfort food, using animal-based ingredients to make a creamy, cheesy dish without traditional pasta.

Ingredients:

2 cups chopped chicken (cooked)
1 cup thick cream
1 1/2 cups cheddar cheese, chopped
1/2 cup cream cheese
Salt and pepper to taste. Preparation Time: 10 minutes
Twenty minutes of cooking time
30 minutes all together

Instruction:

Preheat the oven: Preheat your oven to 350°F (175°C).
Combine Ingredients: In a big bowl, mix shredded chicken, heavy cream, cheddar cheese, cream cheese, salt, and pepper.
Transfer to Baking Dish: Pour the mixture into an oiled baking dish.
Bake: Place in the oven and bake for 20 minutes or until the top is bubbly and golden.
Serve: Allow to cool slightly before serving.

Health Benefits: This dish is rich in protein and fats, with cheeses giving calcium and the chicken offering lean protein.

Dietary Importance: Suitable for a ketogenic diet, this version of mac n' cheese offers comfort food flavor without the carbs, supporting a low-carb, high-fat nutritional regimen.

Introduction: Goat Cheese and Prosciutto Quiche blends the tangy flavors of goat cheese with the rich taste of prosciutto in a deliciously baked egg custard, wrapped in a flaky pastry crust.

Ingredients:

1 premade pie crust (or a homemade low-carb crust for keto diets)
4 eggs
1 cup thick cream
4 ounces goat cheese
4 slices prosciutto, chopped
Add salt and pepper to taste.
Fresh herbs for garnish (such as thyme or basil)
15 minutes to get ready.
Cooking Time: 35 minutes
Total Time: 50 minutes

Instructions:

Preheat the oven: Preheat your oven to 375°F (190°C).
Prepare the Crust: Roll out your pie crust and place it in a pie dish. Crimp the ends as desired.
Whisk Eggs and Cream: In a bowl, mix together eggs and heavy cream. Season with salt and pepper.
Add Fillings: Sprinkle crumbled goat cheese and chopped prosciutto into the pie crust. Pour the egg mixture over the top.
Bake: Bake in the preheated oven for about 35 minutes, or until the custard is set and the top is lightly brown.
Serve: Garnish with fresh herbs before serving. Serve it warm or at room temperature.

Nutritional Benefits: This quiche is rich in proteins and fats, with goat cheese providing a good source of calcium and the egg

Introduction: Lamb with Anchovy Aioli combines the tender, distinct flavor of lamb with a robust, umami-packed anchovy aioli, creating a dish that's both refined and extremely satisfying.

Ingredients:

2 pounds lamb meat chops
Add salt and pepper to taste.
2 tablespoons olive oil
For the Anchovy Aioli:
6 anchovy pieces, minced 1 clove garlic, minced 1/2 cup mayonnaise
Juice of 1 lemon
1 tablespoon olive oil
15 minutes to get ready.
Cooking Time: 15 minutes
30 minutes all together

Instructions:

Prepare Lamb: Season the lamb chops heavily with salt and pepper.
Cook Lamb: Heat olive oil in a pan over medium-high heat. Add lamb chops and cook for about 4-5 minutes on each side for medium-rare, or until done to your taste.
Make Anchovy Aioli: While the lamb cooks, mix minced anchovies, garlic, mayonnaise, lemon juice, and olive oil in a bowl. Stir until smooth.
Serve: Plate the cooked lamb chops and fill with anchovy aioli, or serve the aioli on the side for dipping.

Health Benefits: Lamb is a great source of high-quality protein, essential amino acids, vitamins B12, niacin, zinc, and iron, supporting muscle growth, and cognitive function. Anchovies add healthy fats and omega-3 fatty acids, which are helpful for heart health.

Dietary Importance: This dish is perfect for those following a diet that emphasizes high protein and healthy fats, such as keto or paleo diets.

Lamb Ribs with Chermoula

Introduction: Lamb Ribs with Chermoula bring a North African twist to the table, featuring spiced, aromatic herbs and a vibrant marinade that improves the rich flavors of the lamb.

Ingredients:

3 pounds lamb ribs
Add salt and pepper to taste.
For the Chermoula:
1 cup fresh cilantro, chopped
1 cup fresh parsley, chopped; 3 cloves garlic, minced
1 teaspoon cumin
1 teaspoon paprika
1/2 teaspoon chili powder
1/4 cup olive oil
Juice of 1 lemon
Preparation Time: 20 minutes (plus soaking time)
Cooking Time: 1 hour, 30 minutes
Total Time: About 2 hours

Instructions:

Make Chermoula: In a bowl, mix together cilantro, parsley, garlic, cumin, paprika, chili flakes, olive oil, and lemon juice.
Marinate Ribs: Season the lamb ribs with salt and pepper. Rub the chermoula all over the ribs, then cover and refrigerate for at least 2 hours, ideally overnight.
Preheat the oven: Preheat your oven to 325°F (163°C).

Bake Ribs: Place the marinating ribs on a baking sheet. Cover with foil and bake for about 1.5 hours, or until the meat is soft.
Serve: Remove the paper and broil for a few minutes to crisp up the exterior. Serve hot.

Health Benefits: Lamb ribs are rich in protein, fats, and important nutrients such as zinc and selenium. The herbs and spices in chermoula provide antioxidants and have anti-inflammatory qualities.

Dietary Importance: This flavorful dish fits well into diets that stress whole foods and nutrient-dense ingredients, making it suitable for those focusing on health and wellness through diet.

Pork Belly Fat, Carnivore Chili

Introduction: Pork Belly Fat Carnivore Chili is a hearty, meat-heavy dish that's great for those following a carnivore diet. It's simple yet satisfying, packed with high-fat content to keep you energetic.

Ingredients:

2 pounds pork belly, cut into small cubes
1 pound ground beef
Salt and pepper to taste Water as needed
Ten minutes to get ready.
Cooking Time: 2 hours Total Time: 2 hours, 10 minutes

Ingridients:

Brown Pork Belly: In a big pot, cook the pork belly cubes over medium heat until they start to render fat and become crispy.
Add Ground Beef: Add the ground beef to the pot with the pork belly, season with salt and pepper, and cook until cooked.

Simmer: Once the meats are fully cooked, add enough water to cover the mixture slightly. Reduce the heat to low and let simmer for about 2 hours, stirring occasionally.

Serve: Serve the chili hot, ensuring it's rich and hearty with a high percentage of fats and proteins.

Health Benefits: Pork belly is very high in fat, giving long-lasting energy and essential fatty acids. Ground beef adds high-quality protein and important minerals like iron and zinc.

Dietary Importance: This dish is designed for those on a carnivore diet, focusing on zero carbs and high fat and protein intake to keep energy levels and support muscle health while giving high-quality protein and essential nutrients.

Seafood Alfredo

Introduction: Seafood Alfredo blends tender pieces of seafood with a rich, creamy Alfredo sauce served over pasta. This dish is great for seafood lovers and makes a luxurious meal that's surprisingly easy to prepare.

Ingredients:

8 ounces fettuccine or your choice of pasta
2 sticks of butter
1 cup thick cream
1 cup grated Parmesan cheese
1/2 pound shrimp, peeled and deveined
1/2 pound scallops
Salt and black pepper to taste
1 clove garlic, minced
Fresh parsley, chopped (for garnish)
Ten minutes to get ready.
Twenty minutes of cooking time,

30 minutes all together

Instructions:

Cook Pasta: Cook the pasta according to package directions until al dente. Drain and set away.
Cook Seafood: In a pan, melt one tablespoon of butter over medium heat. Add shrimp and scallops, season with salt and pepper, and cook until opaque, about 2-3 minutes per side. Remove the seafood and set away.
Make Alfredo Sauce: In the same skillet, add the leftover butter and garlic. Sauté for 1 minute. Pour in the heavy cream and bring to a boil. Reduce heat and stir in Parmesan cheese until melted and smooth.
Combine: Return the cooked seafood to the pan with the Alfredo sauce. Stir to coat the fish in the sauce.
Serve: Toss the cooked pasta with the seafood Alfredo sauce. Garnish with chopped parsley and serve quickly.

Health Benefits: This dish is high in protein from the seafood, giving essential amino acids. The heavy cream and Parmesan cheese add calcium and fats, which are important for bone health and give energy.

Dietary Importance: Seafood Alfredo is rich in nutrients important for heart health and muscle maintenance. It's a fulfilling meal that can be part of a balanced diet when eaten in moderation.

Salmon with Cream Cheese Sauce

Introduction: Salmon with Cream Cheese Sauce is an elegant dish that pairs the rich taste of salmon with a smooth, tangy cream cheese sauce. This dish is not only delicious but also packed with omega-3 fatty acids, making it a healthy choice for a polished dinner.

Ingredients:

4 salmon pieces, about 6 ounces each
Salt and black pepper to taste
2 tablespoons olive oil
1/2 cup cream cheese
1/4 cup milk
1 tablespoon fresh dill, chopped
1 teaspoon lemon juice
1 tablespoon lemon juice
Ten minutes to get ready.
Cooking Time: 15 minutes
25 minutes all together

Instructions:

Prepare Salmon: Season salmon pieces with salt and pepper.
Cook Salmon: Heat olive oil in a pan over medium heat. Add salmon pieces, skin-side down, and cook for about 6-7 minutes on each side or until cooked through and easily flaked with a fork.
Make Cream Cheese Sauce: In a small pot, heat cream cheese and milk over low heat. Stir until the cream cheese is melted and the sauce is smooth. Add dill, lemon peel, and lemon juice. Stir to combine.
Serve: Place cooked salmon on plates. Pour the cream cheese sauce over the salmon. Serve quickly.

Nutritional Benefits: Salmon is a superb source of omega-3 fatty acids, which are necessary for brain function and cardiovascular health. Cream cheese adds a good amount of iron and protein.

Dietary Importance: This dish supports a heart-healthy diet and can help in lowering inflammation due to the high omega-3 content in salmon. It's perfect for those looking to maintain a balanced diet with a focus on health and well-being.

Conclusion

As you turn the last pages of this book, it's my hope that the recipes you've found have increased your appreciation for wholesome, tasty meals as well as encouraged culinary experimentation. Every recipe, created to tantalize your taste buds and supply vital nutrition.

Consider food as a deep statement of culture, health, and inventiveness as well as a source of nutrition. The meals you've seen on these pages are invitations to celebrate the variety of foods and the countless opportunities they offer, not merely recipes. Setting a table for one or throwing a feast for many, cooking, and sharing food are very intimate and social activities.

A culinary adventure extends outside the kitchen. It's an adventure that pushes you to use items for their health advantages as well as their flavor. Every dish in this book challenges you to think about what goes on your plate and how it could improve your general health and well-being. Choosing to cook and eat this way means honoring your body and mind.

As you go through these dishes, never forget that your kitchen is an innovation lab. Try new methods, substitutes, and don't be afraid to modify the recipes to fit your dietary requirements and preferences. One of the nicest things about cooking is its adaptability; the more you prepare, the more proficient and self-assured you will get.

Though your trip through the pages of this book may come to an end, cooking never ends. Every dinner presents a chance to nourish your spirit as well as your body. Get guests to enjoy the cooking process, sample your culinary creations, and take pride in the meals you offer.

When a meal doesn't come out as planned, keep in mind that every error is a teaching moment. Like life, cooking has many unanticipated twists and turns. Graciously and humorously welcome these times, and never be afraid to try again.

Ultimately, I hope this book continues to be a reliable tool in your kitchen, a travel companion for your culinary explorations, and a reminder of the happiness that comes from cooking. To a lifetime of delicious discoveries, to the pleasures of shared meals, and to your further study of the culinary arts.

I appreciate you including this recipe collection in your culinary adventure. There are many more delicious and nourishing dinners to come. Good cooking!